Lecture Notes in Artificial Intelligence   10526

Subseries of Lecture Notes in Computer Science

U Kang · Ee-Peng Lim
Jeffrey Xu Yu · Yang-Sae Moon (Eds.)

Trends and Applications in Knowledge Discovery and Data Mining

PAKDD 2017 Workshops, MLSDA, BDM, DM-BPM
Jeju, South Korea, May 23, 2017
Revised Selected Papers

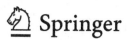 Springer

Editors
U Kang
Seoul National University
Seoul
Korea (Republic of)

Ee-Peng Lim
School of Information Systems
Singapore Management University
Singapore
Singapore

Jeffrey Xu Yu
Chinese University of Hong Kong
Hong Kong
China

Yang-Sae Moon (iD)
Kangwon National University
Chuncheon
Korea (Republic of)

ISSN 0302-9743   ISSN 1611-3349   (electronic)
Lecture Notes in Artificial Intelligence
ISBN 978-3-319-67273-1   ISBN 978-3-319-67274-8   (eBook)
DOI 10.1007/978-3-319-67274-8

Library of Congress Control Number: 2017955721

LNCS Sublibrary: SL7 – Artificial Intelligence

Printed on acid-free paper

This Springer imprint is published by Springer Nature
The registered company is Springer International Publishing AG
The registered company address is: Gewerbestrasse 11, 6330 Cham, Switzerland

Preface

This edited volume contains selected papers from the four workshops that were held on May 23, 2017, in Jeju, South Korea. These workshops were run in conjunction with the 21st Pacific-Asia Conference on Knowledge Discovery and Data Mining (PAKDD 2017), a leading international conference in the areas of data mining and knowledge discovery. The four workshops are: Workshop on Machine Learning for Sensory Data Analysis (MLSDA), Workshop on Biologically Inspired Data-Mining Techniques (BDM), Pacific Asia Workshop on Intelligence and Security Informatics (PAISI), and Workshop on Data Mining in Business Process Management (DM-BPM). The aim of these workshops was to provide forums for discussing research topics related to emerging data mining theories and real-life applications, where knowledge discovery was found to be necessary and/or useful.

In the PAKDD 2017 workshops, each submitted paper was rigorously reviewed by at least two Program Committee members. Although many papers were worthy of publication, only 26 regular papers could be accepted for presentation at the workshops and publication in this volume. The general quality of submissions was high and the competition was tough. We would like to thank all the authors who submitted their papers on many exciting and important research topics to the PAKDD workshops. We thank the workshop organizers for their tremendous effort and valuable time to make the workshops possible. We also thank all the workshop participants and presenters for attending these workshops. It is our hope that the workshops will provide a lasting platform for disseminating the latest research results and practice of data-mining approaches and applications.

These workshops would not have been possible without the help of many colleagues. We would like to thank the Program Committee members for their invaluable review time and comments. Given the extremely tight review schedule, their effort to complete the review reports before the deadline was greatly appreciated. In addition, we found some reviewers' comments were truly excellent, as good as what is usually found in a survey paper – critical, constructive, and comprehensive. These comments were very helpful for us in selecting the papers.

Thank you all and may the papers collected in the volume inspire your thoughts and research.

July 2017

U Kang
Ee-Peng Lim
Jeffrey Xu Yu
Yang-Sae Moon

BDM 2017 Workshop PC Chairs' Message

For the past few years, biologically inspired data-mining techniques have been intensively used in different data-mining applications such as data clustering, classification, association rule mining, sequential pattern mining, outlier detection, feature selection, and bioinformatics. The techniques include neural networks, evolutionary computation, fuzzy systems, genetic algorithms, ant colony optimization, particle swarm optimization, artificial immune system, culture algorithms, social evolution, and artificial bee colony optimization. A huge increase in the number of papers published in the area has been observed in the past decade. Most of these techniques either hybridize optimization with existing data-mining techniques to speed up the data-mining process or use these techniques as independent data-mining methods to improve the quality of patterns mined from the data.

The aim of the workshop is to highlight the current research related to biologically inspired techniques in different data-mining domains and their implementation in real-life data-mining problems. The workshop provides a platform to researchers from computational intelligence and evolutionary computation and other biologically inspired techniques to get feedback on their work from other data-mining perspectives such as statistical data mining, AI, and machine learning-based data mining.

Following the call for papers, BDM 2017 attracted 17 submissions from seven different countries, where seven of them were accepted after a double-blind review by at least three reviewers. The overall acceptance rate for the workshop was 40%.

The selected papers highlight work in bees swarm optimization for association rules, CFDP algorithms based on shared nearest neighbors, CNN-based sequence labeling, genetic algorithm for interpretable model extraction from decision tree ensembles, self-adaptive weighted extreme learning machine for imbalanced classification problems, estimating word probabilities with neural networks, genetic algorithms for solving the frequent itemsets mining problem, and software vulnerability prediction Web service based on artificial neural networks.

We are thankful to all the help from our colleagues in organizing this workshop. Thanks to the authors who made this workshop possible by submitting their work and responding positively to the changes suggested by our reviewers. We are also thankful to our Program Committee, who dedicated their time and provided us with their valuable suggestions and timely reviews. We wish to express our gratitude to the workshop chairs, who were always available to answer our queries and provided us with everything we needed to put this workshop together.

July 2017

Shafiq Alam
Gillian Dobbie

Organization

Workshop Co-chairs

U Kang	Seoul National University, Korea
Ee-Peng Lim	Singapore Management University, Singapore
Jeffrey Xu Yu	The Chinese University of Hong Kong, Hong Kong, SAR China

MLSDA Workshop (Machine Learning for Sensory Data Analysis)

General Chair

Ashfaqur Rahman	CSIRO, Australia

Program Chair

Jeremiah Deng	University of Otago, New Zealand

Organizing Committee

Jeremiah Deng	University of Otago, New Zealand
Robert Dunne	CSIRO, Australia
Jiuyong Li	University of South Australia, Australia
Bernhard Pfahringer	University of Waikato, New Zealand
Ashfaqur Rahman	CSIRO, Australia

Program Committee

Adnan Al-Anbuky	AUT, New Zealand
Weidong Cai	University of Sydney, Australia
Rachael Cardell-Oliver	UWA, Australia
Paulo De Souza	CSIRO, Australia
Jeremiah Deng	University of Otago, New Zealand
Alberto Elfes	CSIRO, Australia
Clinton Fookes	QUT, Australia
Jia Hu	Hope, UK
Yuan Jiang	Nanjing University, China
Eamonn Keogh	UCR, USA
Irena Koprinska	University of Sydney, Australia
Daniel Lai	University of Victoria, Australia
Christopher Leckie	University of Melbourne, Australia
Ickjai Lee	James Cook, Australia
Ivan Lee	University of South Australia, Australia
Jiuyong Li	University of South Australia, Australia

Craig Lindley	CSIRO, Australia
Ann Nowé	VUB, Belgium
Mariusz Nowostawski	Gjøvik University College, Norway
Paul Pang	Unitec, New Zealand
Matthew Parry	University of Otago, New Zealand
Yonghong Peng	University of Bradford, UK
Bernhard Pfahringer	University of Waikato, New Zealand
Martin Purvis	University of Otago, New Zealand
Ashfaqur Rahman	CISRO, Australia
Daniel Smith	Data61, CSIRO, Australia
James S.C. Tan	(UniSIM), Singapore
Duc A. Tran	University of Massachusetts, USA
Zhiyong Wang	University of Sydney, Australia
Brendon Woodford	University of Otago, New Zealand
Haibo Zhang	University of Otago, New Zealand
Ji Zhang	University of South Queensland, Australia
Jun Zhang	Sun Yat-sen University, China
Zhi-hua Zhou	Nanjing University, China
Xingquan Zhu	UTS, Australia

BDM Workshop (Biologically Inspired Data-Mining Techniques)

Program Co-chairs

| Shafiq Alam Burki | University of Auckland, New Zealand |
| Gillian Dobbie | University of Auckland, New Zealand |

Program Committee

Redda Alhaj	University of Calgary, Canada
Michela Antonelli	University of Pisa, Italy
Stephen Chen	York University, Canada
Emilio Corchado	University of Burgas, Bulgaria
Xiao-Zhi Gao	Aalto University, Finland
Ismail Khalil	Johannes Kepler University, Austria
Ganesh Kumar Venayagamoorthy	Missouri University of Science and Technology, USA
Ming Li	Nanjing University, China
Richi Nayek	QUT, Australia
Kouroush Neshatian	University of Canterbury, New Zealand
Saeed u Rehman	Unitec, Institute of Technology Auckland, New Zealand
Patricia Riddle	University of Auckland, New Zealand
Khalid Saeed	AGH Krakow Poland, Poland
Kamran Shafi	DSARC, UNSW, Australia

Zawar Shah   Whitireia Community Polytechnic, New Zealand
David Taniar   Monash University, Australia
Fatos Xhafa   Universitat Politecnica de Catalunya, Spain
Yanjun Yan   Western Carolina University, USA
Moslem Yousefi   Korea University, Republic of Korea
Lean Yu   Chinese Academy of Sciences (CAS), China

DM-BPM Workshop (Data Mining in Business Process Management)

Workshop Organizers

Marco Comuzzi   UNIST, Korea
Youcef Djenouri   UNIST, Korea
Zineb Habbas   Université de Lorraine, France

Program Committee

Giovanni Acampora   University of Naples Federico II, Italy
Ladjel Belatreche   LIAS/ISAE-ENSMA, Poitiers, France
Massimiliano De Leoni   Eindhoven University of Technology, The Netherlands
Johannes De Smeedt   Katholieke Universiteit Leuven, Belgium
Fabrizio Maggi   University of Tartu, Estonia
Pierluigi Plebani   Politecnico di Milano, Italy
Minseok Song   POSTECH, Korea
Son Tran   CSIRO, Australia
Anna Wilbik   Eindhoven University of Technology, The Netherlands
Peng-Yeng Yin   National Chi Nan University, Taiwan

Contents

DM-BPM

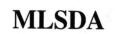

MLSDA

Early Classification of Multivariate Time Series on Distributed and In-Memory Platforms

Vincent S. Tseng[1(✉)], Huai-Shuo Huang[1], Chia-Wei Huang[1], Ping-Feng Wang[2], and Chu-Feng Li[2]

[1] National Chiao Tung University, Hsinchu, Taiwan, Republic of China
vtseng@cs.nctu.edu.tw
[2] Institute for Information Industry, Taipei, Taiwan, Republic of China
{pfwang,chufengli}@iii.org.tw

Abstract. With the popularity of Internet of Things (IOT) applications, various kinds of active sensors are deployed and multivariate time series datasets are generated rapidly. Early classification of multivariate time series is an emerging topic in data mining due to the wide applications in many domains. The unique part of early classification lies in that it uses only earlier part of time series data to reach classification results with the same accuracy as by methods using complete time series information. Although a number of relevant studies have been presented recently, most of them didn't consider the issues of data scale and execution efficiency simultaneously. The main research issue of this paper falls in how to mine interpretable patterns from multivariate time series data, with which effective classification models can be constructed to ensure the accuracy as well as earliness. To take into account the issues of data scale and execution efficiency simultaneously, we explore distributed in-memory computing techniques and multivariate shapelets-based approaches to construct a Spark-based in-memory mining framework to parallelize the feature extraction process. We implement a framework with Multivariate Shapelets Detection (MSD) method as a based example. Through empirical evaluation on various kinds of sensory datasets, the scalability of the framework is evaluated in terms of efficiency while ensuring the same accuracy and reliability in early classification of multivariate time series. This work is the first one to realize multivariate time series early classification on Spark distributed in-memory computing platform, which can serve as a good base for an extension to other time series classification methods based on shapelet feature extraction.

Keywords: Early classification · Multivariate time series · Parallel and distributed computing · Shapelets

1 Introduction

The concept and applications of Internet of Things are getting more and more popular in real-life. Many information products are equipped with various kinds of sensors that can collect data by M2M communications and it brings great convenience to everyone. With the rapid development of IOT techniques, data collection, data storage and data

© Springer International Publishing AG 2017
U Kang et al. (Eds.): PAKDD 2017 Workshops, LNAI 10526, pp. 3–14, 2017.
DOI: 10.1007/978-3-319-67274-8_1

transformation are getting more powerful than before. For example, Smart Meter, Smart Grid and other environmental monitoring equipment are more popular. The frequency of data collection is denser and the variety of collected information is also increased. The data that is collected by a great number of sensors has two major characteristics: (i) They are long sequences of data points. (ii) The continuously measured data points are typically having uniform time intervals. The collected data can be fully represented by time series data format.

Time series analysis is an emerging topic in data mining fields, which has been used in various domains covering medical information, financial market, production management, activity detection and disaster prediction. There are two common ways to analyze time series data. The first one is classical time series classification and the second one is early classification on time series (ECTS). The aim of early classification is naturally different from classical time series classification which only focuses on accuracy without taking earliness into consideration. The tradeoff between accuracy and earliness is an interesting issue in ECTS problem. The goal of ECTS is to make predictions as early as possible and also remains reasonable accuracy. ECTS is often used to detect heart diseases. For example, if we have sample signals from patients who had heart attacks. ECTS can detect and alert before a heart attack happens on new patients. Another example, when an earthquake strikes, if we use time series signals to predict earthquakes, people can prepare and react to it earlier. This may save so many lives. According to the above, the importance of time series early classification cannot be neglected. Besides, time series analysis takes a lot of time to find the patterns in the training phase. For many applications, if the training and predicting can't be done efficiently, it won't be helpful. Hence, efficient computing and mining in big data is a critical issue with new methods requested.

To achieve the goal of real-time training, distributed computing is used in our system. Distributed systems are a group of network computers. Each computer in the group can transfer information and communicate with other computers in the group. There is a coordinator in the group to assign tasks to the others in the group to achieve the goal. The concept of distributed system has the following advantages. (i) If one machine crashes, the system as a whole can still survive. (ii) A distributed system may have more computing power in total than a single mainframe. (iii) It allows many users to access a common database. (iv) It could take less money to increase computing power. In 2006, Apache Hadoop was introduced. Apache Hadoop [20] is an open source platform comes with a distributed file system and other modules like Hadoop YARN [1], Hadoop MapReduce [6], HBase [2], Spark [27], Zookeeper [14], Hive [21], Pig Latin [8] and more. Recently, Spark is more popular than Hadoop because of its in-memory computing characteristics. Spark also supports many languages like Java, Python and Scala. Besides, it is compatible to Hadoop. Based on the above reasons, Spark is used in this research.

There are many existing methods on ECTS. In 2008, [23] uses the feature value to do ECTS problem. The most commonly used method is nearest neighbors [4, 7, 22, 24]. However, the nearest neighbor method can't extract the feature which is interpretable. Recently Many ECTS methods are based on shapelets [5, 16, 25, 26]. Most of them have been proposed to make early predictions on univariate time series. However, to predict accurately, using univariate time series is not enough. Multivariate time series also needs to be considered. Ghalwash and Obradovic [9, 12, 13] started to do research on multivariate time series on ECTS and took multi-shapelets as candidate features (MSD). It can calculate the distance threshold of feature to filter useless patterns. This method is suitable for the homogeneous data and missing value is not allowed in data. To break out the limit of [9], Ghalwash and Obradovic proposed new methods [10, 11] which combined Hidden Markov Model (HMM) and Support Vector Machine (SVM). When it comes to multivariate time series, it takes a lot of time to calculate the distance of shapelets. Lin [15] proposed the method that uses GPU to speed up the computing process. However, the GPU-based methods incur the problem that they can't deal with big data if the memory of GPU is not enough (which is usually the case).

In this paper, to resolve the insufficiency in existing methods as mentioned above, we explore to apply distributed and in-memory computing techniques on a shapelet-based method to enhance the scalability in dealing with large-scale time series data in constructing early classification models for multivariate time series, which could be composed of various kinds of sensory data. We implemented a Spark-based framework to parallelize the feature extraction process of MSD method to explore the aim as mentioned above. The framework was evaluated by using various kinds of sensory datasets from different application domains. The result presents the performance of our framework compared to the single-threaded version of the MSD method on multivariate time series early classification in dimensions of scalability, accuracy and reliability. This work is the first one to realize multivariate time series early classification on Spark distributed in-memory computing platform. Our framework defined a new way to speed up the training process of multivariate time series early classification and can serve as a good base for an extension to other time series classification methods based on shapelet feature extraction.

The remainder of this paper is organized as follow. Section 2 introduces some basic concepts and related works of ECTS. We then explain our framework in Sect. 3. Section 4 will explain how we did the experiment and show the results of our experiments. At last, we will have a conclusion for this paper and talk about the future works.

2 Preliminaries and Related Work

2.1 Preliminaries

In this section, we introduce the definitions and properties of multivariate time series, shapelet and other objects.

Definition 1 (Time series). A time series $T = \{t_1, t_2, \cdots, t_L\}$ of length L, len(T) = L, is defined as a sequence of L real values. A subsequence of a time series T is defined as $s = \{t_i, t_{i+1}, \cdots, t_L\}$, s ⊂ T, is a sampling of contiguous positions of T of length $\ell < L$.

Definition 2 (Distance between subsequences). Given two subsequence s and s′ where len(s) = len(s′) = L, the Euclidean distance between s and t is defined as:

$$\text{dist}(s, s') = \sqrt{\sum_{i=1}^{L} (s[i] - s'[i])^2}$$

Definition 3 (Distance between subsequence and time series). Given a subsequence s of length ℓ and a time series t of length L, the distance between s and t is defined as the minimum distance between s and all the subsequences of t with the same length. The distance between s and t is computed as:

$$\text{dist}(s, t) = \min_{\forall i \in \{1,2,...,L-\ell+1\}} dist(s, t_i)$$

where t_i is a subsequence of t of length ℓ starting from position i.

Definition 4 (Multivariate time series). An N-dimensional multivariate time series (MTS) of length L is defined as $T = \{T^1, T^2, \cdots, T^N\}$ where T^j is a time series that represents the jth dimension of T. Each multivariate time series is associated with a class label $c \in C$ where C is a finite set of class labels. A dataset D is a collection of M pairs $\{(T_1, c_1), (T_2, c_2), \cdots, (T_i, c_i), \cdots, (T_M, c_M)\}$ where T_i is a multivariate time series and c_i is its class label.

Definition 5 (N-dimensional shapelet). An N-dimensional shapelet (N-shapelet) is defined as $f = (s, \ell, \Delta, c_f)$. The vector $s = [s^1, s^2, \cdots, s^N]$ where s^j is a time series that represents the jth dimension of the shapelet. ℓ is the length of the shapelet. The distance threshold $\Delta = [\delta^1, \delta^2, \cdots, \delta^N]$. Finally c_f is a class label.

Definition 6 (Distance between N-shapelet and multivariate time series). Given an N-shapelet f and an N-dimensional multivariate time series T. The distance between them is defined as:

$$\text{dist}(s, T) = [dist(s^1, T^1), dist(s^2, T^2), ..., dist(s^N, T^N)]$$

where $dist(s^j, T^j)$ is defined in Definition 3.

2.2   Related Works

The very first research on time series early classification is done by Rodriguez et al. [19]. This research uses the prefix of time series to predict, but it did not optimize the earliness of predictions. In the year 2008, Xing et al. [23] applied a feature based method on sequence early classification. Unfortunately, it can only be used on symbolic sequences, instead of real value time series. Meanwhile, according to the characteristic of the algorithm, it is hard to be applied to multivariate time series. Many research works such as [4, 7, 22, 24] were extended from the nearest neighbor approach. However, these methods cannot extract features with interpretability. Recently, the concept of shapelet emerged [16, 17, 26] and has been used as features in time series early classification.

All of the methods above can only be applied on univariate time series. When it comes to multivariate time series, shapelet-based methods have to be modified. In 2012, Ghalwash et al. [9] proposed a shapelet-based method for early classification on multivariate time series (MSD). MSD was one of the first methods that applied N-dimensional shapelet on early classification. Same as all the other shapelet-based methods, feature extraction process in MSD consumes a tremendous amount of time. It's very inefficient and hard to be applied for real word datasets.

3 Methodology

3.1 Multivariate Shapelets Detection

The Multivariate Shapelets Detection method is proposed in [9]. Figure 1 shows the whole algorithm of MSD in pseudocode. It contains three major parts: (I) Feature extraction, (II) Shapelet pruning and (III) Classification. In this section, we will explain these parts in details.

```
Input: A training dataset D of M multivariate time series; minL; maxL
Output: A list of multivariate shapelets
1.  for each time series T ∈ D do // T is a time series of length L
2.    for l ←minL to maxL do //for each shapelet length
3.      for k ←1 to L - 1 + 1 do //for each starting position
4.        RowDist = ShapeletDist(k,l,Dist)
5.        ComputeThreshold (f_lk, RowDist)
6.        ComputeUtilityScore (f_lk)
7.        Add(f_lk, ShapeletList )
8.  PruneShapelets(ShapeletList )
9.  return ShapeletList
```

Fig. 1. The algorithm of Multivariate Shapelets Detection (MSD) method [9] for multivariate time series.

3.1.1 Feature Extraction

All the N-dimensional shapelets $f = (s, \ell, \Delta, c_f)$ are extracted from training dataset D by using sliding window techniques. The MSD method will extract a subsequence from each dimension on every training data. In $s = [s^1, s^2, \cdots, s^N]$, s^j is the extracted subsequence from the jth dimension of training time series. To calculate distance threshold of a shapelet, the method order two multidimensional distance $d_1 = [d_1^1, d_1^2, \ldots, d_1^N]$ and $d_2 = [d_2^1, d_2^2, \ldots, d_2^N]$ according to the following rule:

$$d_1 < d_2 \text{ iff } d_1^j < d_2^j \ \forall j = 1 \ldots N$$

In the above equation, all N dimensions of d_1 need to be less than all corresponding dimensions of d_2, that might lead to over fitting. To prevent overfitting, the MSD method relaxes and redefines the equation to the following criteria:

$$d_1 <_{Perc} d_2 \; iff \; d_1^{a_j} < d_2^{a_j} \; \forall j = 1 \ldots Perc \times N$$

where Perc $\in (0, 1]$ determines the percentage of dimensions used to compare.

The feature extraction algorithm for multivariate shapelets is similar to the algorithm showed in Fig. 1. It takes 3 for-loops to extract all multivariate shapelets. For each shapelet candidate, the algorithm computes the distance vector of length N. After distance calculation, MSD method finds the distances matrix with dimensions N × M between a multivariate shapelet and all time series where M is the number of time series. The process of finding shapelet for each time series is independent. This is one reason for us to parallel this part in the Distributed Feature Extraction section.

Then, it takes a multivariate shapelet f and the distance matrix as input and computes the distance threshold of f based on information gain [9]. In the end, the method returns the multivariate threshold $\Delta = [\delta^1, \delta^2, \cdots, \delta^N]$ of multivariate shapelet f that maximize its information gain.

After feature extraction, there are too many shapelets to make a precise and efficient classification. In the MSD method, they also provide a feature selection method that prunes the candidate shapelets.

3.1.2   Shapelet Pruning

The shapelet pruning step of MSD method is based on weighted information gain. First, they define the earliness between a shapelet $f = (s, \ell, \Delta, c_f)$ and a multivariate time series T as

$$EML(f, T) = \min_{i \in \{1,2,\ldots,L-l+1\}} dist(s, h_i) \le \Delta$$

where h_i is the subsequence of length ℓ of T starting from the ith time point. A better shapelet can classify a time series with lower EML. The weighted information gain of the shapelet is computed as follows [9]:

1. Compute the distance between the multivariate shapelet $f = (s, \ell, \Delta, c_f)$ and every time series T_i in the dataset.
2. Split the dataset D into two datasets D_L and D_R such that D_L contains all time series where $dist(f, T_i) \le \Delta$ and D_R contains all time series where $dist(f, T_i) \ge \Delta$.
3. For each time series T in the dataset D_L, if Class(T) = c_f, then T is weighted by EML(f, T). Otherwise, the time series is weighted by 1.
4. Compute M_L as the weighted count of the number of time series in the dataset D_L and M_R is the size of the dataset D_R.
5. Compute the weighted information gain using the following equation

$$IG = Entropy - \frac{M_L}{M} E_L - \frac{M_R}{M} E_R$$

Once the weighted information gains for all multivariate shapelets have been computed, the method sorts the shapelets in descending order by their weighted information gain. The pruning algorithm takes the shapelet from the highest gain and removes all training samples that are covered by this shapelet. The method then takes the next highest ranked shapelet. If the shapelet covers some training samples, the samples are removed and the shapelet is selected. If not, the shapelet is discarded and the algorithm proceeds to the next one. It stops when all training samples are removed.

3.1.3   Classification

The classification process can start when the length of test time series is greater or equal to the length of the shortest shapelet. From all shapelets that are shorter than the test time series, the highest-ranked one is chosen to match the test time series. If matched, the time series is predicted. Otherwise, the next highest-ranked is tried. If none of the shapelets matches the test time series, the method reads the next time stamp into the test time series. As the length of test time series growth, more shapelets can be tried when matching. If the test time series reaches its max length and none of the shapelets covers it, the method marks the time series as not-classified example.

3.2   Distributed Feature Extraction

In order to make the MSD method more efficient, we parallelize the distance calculation process in the early phase of feature extraction since it is the most time-consuming part in the whole method. Figure 2 shows the parallel version of the method in pseudocode.

```
Input: A training dataset D of M multivariate time series; minL; maxL
Output: A list of multivariate shapelets
1.  parallel for each time series T ∈ D do //T is a time
      series of length L
2.    for l ←minL to maxL do //for each shapelet length
3.      for k ←1 to L - l + 1 do //for each starting po-
        sition
4.        RowDist = ShapeletDist(k,l,Dist)
5.  for each time series T ∈ D do // T is a time series of
      length L
6.    for l ←minL to maxL do //for each shapelet length
7.      for k ←1 to L - l + 1 do //for each starting po-
        sition
8.        ComputeThreshold (f_{lk},RowDist)
9.        ComputeUtilityScore (f_{lk})
10.       Add(f_{lk}, ShapeletList )
11. PruneShapelets(ShapeletList )
12. return ShapeletList
```

Fig. 2. The distributed feature extraction for Multivariate Shapelets Detection (MSD) method.

We implement this parallel version of feature extraction on Spark distributed computing platform. First, we create the resilient distributed dataset (RDD) of training dataset T. After that, we can use a map function to parallelize line 2 to 4 of the algorithm.

4   Experimental Evaluation

4.1   Experiment Setup

We use several real datasets to evaluate the performance of our framework. All experiments were performed on a cluster of six computers and each computer has the same Intel Pentium(R) CPU @ 3.2 GHz * 2 with 15.6 GB of memory. The algorithm is implemented in JAVA. Our operating system is Ubuntu 14.04.

4.2   Data Set

The experiments were performed on several real datasets: robot execution failures dataset [3], and ozone level detection dataset [3], ECG dataset [18]. Each multivariate time series dataset is representing a different domain of sensory data.

There are five datasets in the robot execution failures, each of them defines a different problem: failures in approach to grasping position (Rob1), failures in transfer of an object (Rob2), position of an object after a transfer failure (Rob3), failures in approach to ungrasping position (Rob4), failures in motion with an object (Rob5). All of these datasets had no missing feature value and captured the information about 3-axis force and torque from sensors. Each failure instance is characterized in term of 15 samples collected at regular time intervals starting immediately after failure detection. In this experiment, we choose Rob4 to do the experiment. It is a multiclass dataset with 21% normal, 62% collision, 18% obstruction.

Each instance on the ozone level detects dataset recorded two time series of 24 time points of temperature and wind speed. The time series represents one day from January 1, 1999 to December 31, 2004. The dataset contains 2361 instances including 2290 normal days and 71 ozone days after filtering the days without any information.

The ECG dataset used two electrodes to collect heartbeat. Each heartbeat is described by a multivariate time series with a label of normal or abnormal. The abnormal heartbeats are representative of a cardiac pathology known as a supraventricular premature beat (SVPB). There are 200 instances in the dataset, 133 instances are normal and 67 instances are abnormal. The length of ECG is from 39 to 152. Table 1 shows the information of the dataset in the experiment.

Table 1.   Information on different datasets

	Number of training data	Number of testing data	Min length	Max length	Number of variates
Rob4	80	37	15	15	1
OZONE	1651	710	24	24	2
ECG	139	61	39	152	2

4.3   Experiment Result

We randomly split the data into training data (70%) and testing data (30%). In this experiment, we focus on execution time. As shown in Fig. 3, the x-axis represents the number of Spark executors and the y-axis represents training time. The dashed line is the training time without using Spark. As we can see, if we use only one executor, the training time is longer than original algorithm due to communication overhead costs in Spark. However, when we use more than two executors, the training time decrease and eventually become less than the original algorithm. We can also see that when more executors are used, the gradient of speed up slows down. It follows the Amdahl's law. It means that the ideal speedup is bounded by the ratio of parallelism. No matter how we increase the number of processors, the acceleration is limited.

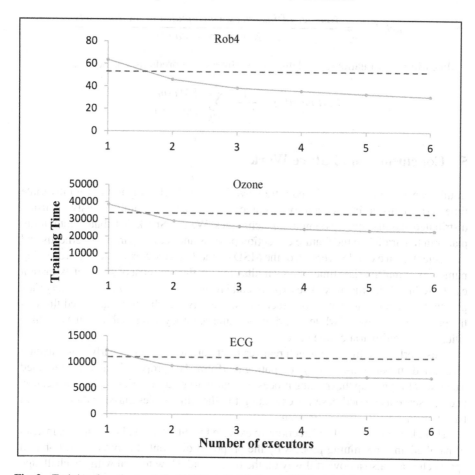

Fig. 3.   Training time (in second) of MSD on Rob4, Ozone, ECG with different numbers of Spark executors. The dashed line is the training time without using Spark.

Table 2 shows the match rate, accuracy and earliness of each dataset. The result shows MSD with Spark could do the same as the result of MSD without using Spark.

Table 2. Result of different datasets

	Match rate	Accuracy	Earliness
Rob4	0.864	0.687	6.2
OZONE	0.985	0.797	4
ECG	0.737	0.666	44

Match rate shows the percentage of instances matching to the shapelets. It is defined as below.

$$Match\ Rate = \frac{Number\ of\ instances\ which\ match\ to\ the\ shapelets}{Number\ of\ instances}$$

In earliness evaluations, we define the earliness of a prediction as below.

$$Earliness(\%) = \frac{1}{D_{test}} \sum_{mt \in D_{test}} \frac{EMT(mt)}{len(mt)}$$

5   Conclusion and Future Work

In this paper, we have introduced a framework for early classification of multivariate time series considering scalability, accuracy and reliability simultaneously by using distributed and in-memory computing techniques. We use Spark distributed computing platform to parallelize the feature extraction process and reduce parallel overheads and implemented an extended version of the MSD method as a base example. By processing numerous of multivariate time series simultaneously, the time cost of shapelet extraction can be reduced significantly. The experimental results on various kinds of sensory data present the effects and degree of execution scalability which can be achieved through the proposed framework while ensuring the same accuracy and reliability in early classification of multivariate time series.

This work is the first one which realizes multivariate time series early classification on Spark distributed in-memory computing platform. The proposed framework defined a new way to speed up the training process of multivariate time series early classification and can serve as a good base for extending to other time series classification methods based on shapelet feature extraction.

There leave some further directions to explore for future work. For example, instead of parallelizing the mining process by the proposed distributed approach, GPU-based approaches are also a powerful way on the other hand. How to deal with the challenge in face of big data under constrained memory (which is usually the case) of GPU-based methods will be an interesting research topic. The combination of distributed in-memory approaches like the proposed framework with the GPU-based approach will be another even more promising direction.

Acknowledgement. This study was conducted under the "Complex Event Processing System" project of the Institute for Information Industry which is subsidized by the Ministry of Economic Affairs of the Republic of China.

References

1. Apache Hadoop. http://hadoop.apache.org/
2. Apache HBase. http://hbase.apache.org/
3. Bache, K., Lichman, M.: UCI machine learning repository (2013)
4. Bregón, A., Simón, M.A., Rodríguez, J.J., Alonso, C., Pulido, B., Moro, I.: Early fault classification in dynamic systems using case-based reasoning. In: Marín, R., Onaindía, E., Bugarín, A., Santos, J. (eds.) CAEPIA 2005. LNCS, vol. 4177, pp. 211–220. Springer, Heidelberg (2006). doi:10.1007/11881216_23
5. Dachraoui, A., Bondu, A., Cornuéjols, A.: Early classification of time series as a non myopic sequential decision making problem. In: Appice, A., Rodrigues, P., Santos Costa, V., Soares, C., Gama, J., Jorge, A. (eds.) ECML PKDD 2015. LNCS, vol. 4177, pp. 433–447. Springer, Cham (2015). doi:10.1007/978-3-319-23528-8_27
6. Dean, J., Ghemawat, S.: MapReduce: simplified data processing on large clusters. Commun. ACM **51**(1), 107–113 (2008)
7. Ding, H., Trajcevski, G., Scheuermann, P., Wang, X., Keogh, E.: Querying and mining of time series data: experimental comparison of representations and distance measures. Proc. VLDB Endow. **1**(2), 1542–1552 (2008)
8. Gates, A.F., Natkovich, O., Chopra, S., Kamath, P., Narayanamurthy, S.M., Olston, C., Reed, B., Srinivasan, S., Srivastava, U.: Building a high-level dataflow system on top of Map-Reduce: the Pig experience. Proc. VLDB Endow. **2**(2), 1414–1425 (2009)
9. Ghalwash, M.F., Obradovic, Z.: Early classification of multivariate temporal observations by extraction of interpretable shapelets. BMC Bioinform. **13**(1), 1 (2012)
10. Ghalwash, M.F., Ramljak, D., Obradović, Z.: Early classification of multivariate time series using a hybrid HMM/SVM model. In: 2012 IEEE International Conference on Bioinformatics and Biomedicine (BIBM), pp. 1–6. IEEE, October 2012
11. Ghalwash, M.F., Radosavljevic, V., Obradovic, Z.: Extraction of interpretable multivariate patterns for early diagnostics. In: 2013 IEEE 13th International Conference on Data Mining (ICDM), pp. 201–210. IEEE, December 2013
12. Ghalwash, M.F., Radosavljevic, V., Obradovic, Z.: Utilizing temporal patterns for estimating uncertainty in interpretable early decision making. In: Proceedings of the 20th ACM SIGKDD International Conference on Knowledge Discovery and Data Mining, pp. 402–411. ACM, August 2014
13. He, G., Duan, Y., Peng, R., Jing, X., Qian, T., Wang, L.: Early classification on multivariate time series. Neurocomputing **149**, 777–787 (2015)
14. Junqueira, F.P., Reed, B.C.: The life and times of a zookeeper. In: Proceedings of the 28th ACM Symposium on Principles of Distributed Computing, p. 4. ACM, August 2009
15. Lin, Y.F., Chen, H.H., Tseng, V.S., Pei, J.: Reliable early classification on multivariate time series with numerical and categorical attributes. In: Cao, T., Lim, E.P., Zhou, Z.H., Ho, T.B., Cheung, D., Motoda, H. (eds.) PAKDD 2015. LNCS, vol. 9077, pp. 199–211. Springer, Cham (2015). doi:10.1007/978-3-319-18038-0_16
16. Lines, J., Davis, L.M., Hills, J., Bagnall, A.: A shapelet transform for time series classification. In: Proceedings of the 18th ACM SIGKDD International Conference on Knowledge Discovery and Data Mining, pp. 289–297. ACM, August 2012

17. Mueen, A., Keogh, E., Young, N.: Logical-shapelets: an expressive primitive for time series classification. In: Proceedings of the 17th ACM SIGKDD International Conference on Knowledge Discovery and Data Mining, pp. 1154–1162. ACM, August 2011

18. Olszewski, R.T.: Generalized feature extraction for structural pattern recognition in time-series data (No. CMU-CS-01-108). Carnegie-Mellon University Pittsburgh, PA School of Computer Science (2001)

19. Rodríguez, J.J., Alonso, C.J., Boström, H.: Boosting interval based literals. Intell. Data Anal. **5**(3), 245–262 (2001)

20. Shvachko, K., Kuang, H., Radia, S., Chansler, R.: The Hadoop distributed file system. In: 2010 IEEE 26th Symposium on Mass Storage Systems and Technologies (MSST), pp. 1–10. IEEE, May 2010

21. Thusoo, A., Sarma, J.S., Jain, N., Shao, Z., Chakka, P., Anthony, S., Liu, H., Wyckoff, P., Murthy, R.: Hive: a warehousing solution over a map-reduce framework. Proc. VLDB Endow. **2**(2), 1626–1629 (2009)

22. Xi, X., Keogh, E., Shelton, C., Wei, L., Ratanamahatana, C.A.: Fast time series classification using numerosity reduction. In: Proceedings of the 23rd International Conference on Machine Learning, pp. 1033–1040. ACM, June 2006

23. Xing, Z., Pei, J., Dong, G., Philip, S.Y.: Mining sequence classifiers for early prediction. In: SDM, pp. 644–655, April 2008

24. Xing, Z., Pei, J., Philip, S.Y.: Early prediction on time series: a nearest neighbor approach. In: IJCAI, pp. 1297–1302, July 2009

25. Xing, Z., Pei, J., Philip, S.Y., Wang, K.: Extracting interpretable features for early classification on time series. In: SDM, vol. 11, pp. 247–258, April 2011

26. Ye, L., Keogh, E.: Time series shapelets: a new primitive for data mining. In: Proceedings of the 15th ACM SIGKDD International Conference on Knowledge Discovery and Data Mining, pp. 947–956. ACM, June 2009

27. Zaharia, M., Chowdhury, M., Das, T., Dave, A., Ma, J., McCauley, M., Franklin, M.J., Shenker, S., Stoica, I.: Resilient distributed datasets: a fault-tolerant abstraction for in-memory cluster computing. In: Proceedings of the 9th USENIX Conference on Networked Systems Design and Implementation, p. 2. USENIX Association, April 2012

Behavior Classification of Dairy Cows Fitted with GPS Collars

Robert Dunne[1]([✉]), Dave Henry[2], Richard Rawnsley[3], and Ashfaqur Rahman[1]

[1] Data61, CSIRO, Canberra, Australia
rob.dunne@data61.csiro.au
[2] CSIRO, Agriculture & Food Precision Agriculture & Viticulture,
671 Sneydes Road, Werribee, VIC 3030, Australia
[3] Tasmanian Institute of Agriculture, Hobart, Australia

Abstract. Precision management systems for livestock offer the potential to monitor and manage animals on an individual basis. A key component of these sensor based systems are the analytical models that automatically translate sensor data into different behavioral categories.

Here we consider the use of GPS data for modelling the behaviour of dairy cows. The performance of this approach is validated across a study involving 24 Holstein-Friesian dairy cows that were each fitted with a GPS unit on a neck collar. The behavior of the cows are classified into 4 general classes: grazing; moving from paddock to paddock; milking; and resting. Using simple rules derived from prior information about the behavior of dairy cows, and information about the layout of the farm, the classification was substantially improved.

The utility of a log of animal behaviour will increase when joined with other data (milk yield, for example) and has the potential to provide useful in animal management, obtained at little cost.

Keywords: Behavior classification · Machine learning · Livestock · Precision management · Geographical positioning system, GPS

1 Introduction

Precision management of livestock differs from traditional herd management by tailoring decisions to the individual animal. The aim of precision strategies is to maximize the potential of each animal and ensure resources are allocated efficiently on the farm. An animals behavioral interactions with its physical environment must be continuously monitored for precision management strategies to be successfully implemented. The observed behaviors of each animal must then be linked to management knowledge in areas such as breeding, welfare and nutrition to enable the appropriate action to be taken. For instance, illness can be predicted in cattle when there is a reduction in the level of social interaction or rumination and feed intake [4,13]. Furthermore, other behavioral changes have been shown to be indicative of when cattle are: lame [10]; in estrus [1,2]; in pain [7]; or under heat stress [3].

U Kang et al. (Eds.): PAKDD 2017 Workshops, LNAI 10526, pp. 15–25, 2017.
DOI: 10.1007/978-3-319-67274-8_2

Sensors and digital technologies are becoming an important enabler for precision livestock management. Sensor based monitoring systems offer the potential for continuous and autonomous monitoring of cattle without the need for human involvement. Such systems generally consist of a sensor or suite of sensors that are fitted to each animal and a model that uses the sensor data to infer the animals behavior. Commercial monitoring systems classify the basic behaviors of a cow, but most importantly, compare the classified behaviors to rules regarding the animals expected or normal behavior in order to alert to potential management issues [1,2,4].

Here we consider the use of GPS data for modelling the behaviour of dairy cows. The performance of this approach is validated across a study involving 24 Holstein-Friesian dairy cows that were each fitted with a GPS unit on a collar around their neck.

We have GPS data, collected every 10 s, on the 24 cows over a 14 day period from 27/11/2012 to 10/12/2012. The cows are part of a single herd of 300 animals on a farm located in the north-east of Tasmania.

In some instances (111 animal days) the GPS record is complete for an animal over a 24 h period. In others (136 animal days) it is only a partial record that may or may not contain usable information. We have behavioral data collected by observers for brief periods during the 14 day period. However, the data was found to cover too brief an interval, was often recorded at very short intervals (2 s) and covered too many activities (chewing, resting with head up, etc.) to be usefully matched to GPS records.

Instead we have explored several other options. We have investigated unsupervised segmentation techniques that have been applied to GPS trajectories collected from wild animals [6]. These are shown to have some utility in interpreting the trajectories.

We have also investigated classifying a limited number of trajectories by eye, relying on domain knowledge of the behavior of diary cows. We can then use these trajectories as data to train a classifier. Hence we are automating a process of information extraction that could be done more laboriously by the farmer.

In addition we have used a number of heuristic rules to improve the classification. We find that, using a classifier and several simple heuristic rules, it is possible to classify the animals behaviour into 4 broad classes, that is: milking (at the milking sheds); moving from paddock to paddock; grazing; and resting.

2   Methods

2.1   Cattle Collar Instrumentation

The behavior monitoring collars [12] fitted to the dairy cows were comprised of a 20-channel GPS receiver chip, an active GPS antennae, a microcontroller and 915 MHz transceiver, a 4 GB micro SD card for data storage and a Honeywell HMC6343 compass module containing a 3-axis MEMS accelerometer and a 3-axis magneto-resistive (magnetometer) sensor. The compass module of the behavior monitoring collars acted as an Inertial Measurement Unit (IMU).

The IMU was ignored as the focus of this particular study was upon classifying cattle behavior using the GPS. The effective battery life was approximately 14 days. After retrieval of the collars at the end of the data collection period, the memory storage cards were removed and the data downloaded and converted from binary format.

2.2 Segmenting a Trajectory into Segments Characterized by a Homogeneous Behaviour 1

Calenge (2006) describes an approach to the segmentation of movement data into homogeneous segments. The method relies on a Bayesian partitioning of a sequence and was originally developed for partitioning DNA sequences [8].

Suppose that the steps, the distances between successive locations, have been independently generated by Gaussian distributions, with different means corresponding to different behaviours. We generate $d = 1, \ldots, D$ models with different means. Based on these *a priori* models we estimate both the number and the extent of the segments building up the trajectory.

Given an optimal k-partition of the trajectory, if the ith step of the trajectory belongs to the segment k predicted by the model d, then either the move $i - 1$ belongs to the same segment, in which case the segment containing $i - 1$ is predicted by d, or the move $i - 1$ belongs to a different segment, and the other $(k-1)$ segments together constitute an optimal $(k-1)$ partition of the trajectory $[1 : (i - 1)]$.

Calenge (2006) uses a range of equally spaced means across the observed range of the steps, with a common variance. We suspect that the means of the behaviors we are interested in are not equally spaced and have differing variances so we fit a mixture of 4 Gaussians using the EM algorithm. For the trajectory of animal 6 on day 2 (Fig. 1) we get the 4 distributions, plotted in Fig. 2.

Figure 3 shows the sequential step lengths. The mean of the Gaussian that best models each segment is shown by a horizontal bar. Figure 4 shows the segmented trajectory.

2.3 Segmenting a Trajectory into Segments Characterized by a Homogeneous Behaviour 2

Calenge [6] also describes a method of

- calculating the residence time for each location on the trajectory;
- use the method of Lavielle [9] to partition the trajectory.

The method of Lavielle finds the best segmentation of a time series, given that it is built by K segments. It searches the possible segmentations for one in which the difference between the observed trajectory and the model is minimized. Let Y_{t_i} be the value of the variable (e.g. residence time, although other variables are possible) at time t_i. We suppose that the data have been generated by the following model:

$$Y_{t_i} = \mu_{t_i} + \sigma_{t_i}\epsilon_{t_i}$$

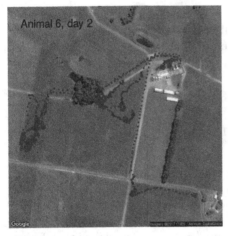

Fig. 1. The trajectory of animal 6 on day 2.

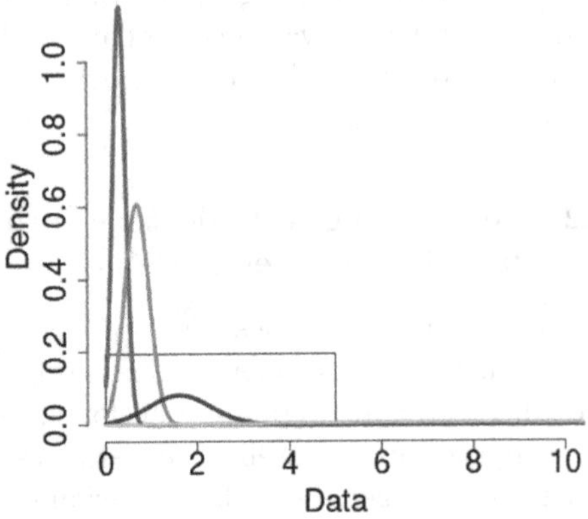

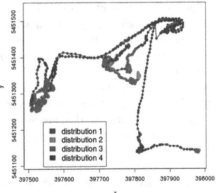

Fig. 2. The mixture of Gaussians fitted to the distances for Animal 6, day 2.

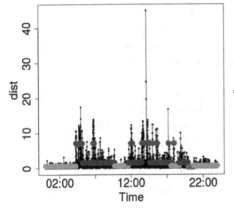

Fig. 3. The sequential step lengths. The mean of the Gaussian that best models each segment is shown by a horizontal bar.

Fig. 4. The segmented path for animal 6 on day 2 using the method of Sect. 2.2.

where μ_{t_i} and σ_{t_i} are the mean and standard deviation of Y_{t_i}. ϵ_{t_i} is a sequence of zero mean random variables with unit variance, not necessarily independent.

We use the most general model, assuming that (writing t_i as i) μ_i and σ_i can both vary between segments, but are constant within a segment. For a given partition of the series built by K segments with known limits, the following function can be used to measure the discrepancy between the observed trajectory

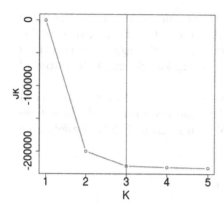
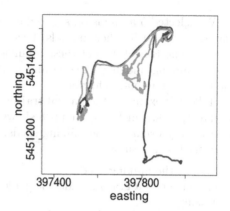

Fig. 5. A plot of $J(K)$ versus K indicates that 3 segments will minimize $J(K)$. Subsequent segments add little to the reduction in the value of $J(K)$.

Fig. 6. The segmented path using $K = 4$ with the method of Lavielle [9].

and the model:

$$J_k(Y) = \sum_{k=1}^{K} G_k(Y_{i,i \in k}),$$

where

$$G_k(Y_{i,i \in k}) = \frac{1}{n(k)} \log \left(\frac{1}{n(k)} \sum_{i=t_1^k}^{t_{n(k)}^k} (Y_i - \bar{Y}_k)^2 \right)$$

where $n(k)$ is the number of steps in segment k. The method of Lavielle uses a dynamic programming algorithm to find the best segmentation of the trajectory, i.e. the segmentation for which $J_k(Y)$ is minimized. The optimal number of segments K is a parameter in the model and [9] suggest plotting $J(K)$ versus K to see if there is a clear "break" at an optimal value of K. Figure 5 shows this plot for animal 6, day 2, and Fig. 6 shows the resulting segmentation into 3 classes.

2.4 Classification Based on Derived Variables from Fixed Time Segments

We take the 10s spaced location data and summarize it to longer segments. We derive a number of variables from each segment:

- the distance between the staring point and the end point of the segment;
- the total distance travelled in the segment;
- the max movement in any 10s segment; and
- the maximum difference in movements between 10s segments.

We selected 5 animals on single days as the training data set (animal 21 on day 1, etc.) and 5 other animals/days as the test data set (animal 6 on day 1, etc.). The trajectories of these animals were manually segmented into the 4 classes milking; moving, grazing and resting, using knowledge of the layout of the farm and animal behaviour.

Take, for example, the partial trajectory (from 07:00 to 17:00) of animal 21 on day 1, shown in Fig. 7. Figure 8 shows the same trajectory as distance from an arbitrary origin at the milking sheds. We can segment it into the following sequential behaviours;

- time at the milking shed.
- movement to a grazing paddock (paddock 1);
- grazing;
- movement to the milking sheds;
- time at the milking shed;
- movement to a grazing paddock (paddock 2);
- grazing.

This divides the animals behavior into 3 classes: milking; moving; and grazing, as shown by the trajectory color in Figs. 7 and 8. For this trajectory there was no resting class.

The derived variables were calculated and a linear discriminant analysis was used to classify the segments. The classification was then tested on the 5 test animals. Segment length of 2, 5 and 10 min were tried with overall classification accuracies of 0.58, 0.58 and 0.61.

See Fig. 9 which shows the classified trajectory for one of the test animals (animal 6 on day 1) using segments of 10 min duration.

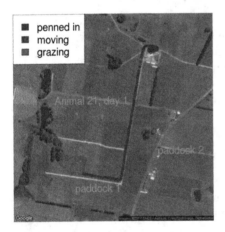

Fig. 7. Animal 21, day 1. Segmented into three classes: penned in (at the milking shed); moving and grazing on the basis of knowledge about the farms practice.

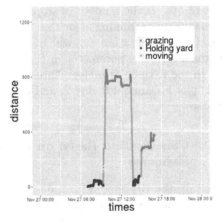

Fig. 8. The trajectory for animal 21, day 1 (Fig. 7) as distance from an arbitrary origin at the milking sheds.

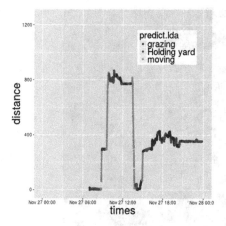 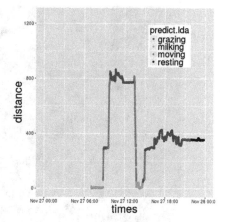

Fig. 9. A classified trajectory for Animal 6, day 1

Fig. 10. A classified trajectory (Fig. 9) after the application of the two heuristic rules.

2.5   Heuristic Rules

We have some prior information about the movement of dairy cows. It is suggested in [5] that:

– grazing occupies about 8 (dairy cows) to 9 (beef cattle) hours a day;
– ruminating occupies about 6 h a day (see also [14]);
– cattle lie down to sleep, ruminate or drowse for nearly half of their day.

In addition we know the layout of the farm and can inspect the typical movements of various animals. This leads us to 2 simple rules:

– the location of the milking shed is fixed and there appears to be no grazing area around it (animals seem to be closely bunched together before milking). We can geo-fence the milking sheds and any time spent in that area can be classed as "milking" time;
– dairy cows do not graze at night. The time between 22:00 and 04:00 (a period when the GPS record shows no more movement than can be attributed to GPS inaccuracy) can be classified as "resting" which includes: resting; sleeping; and ruminating.

Using these simple rules we can improve the behaviour classification. Figure 9 shows a classified trajectory (using the method of Sect. 2.4) and Fig. 10 shows the same classified trajectory after the application of these heuristic rules.

3   Results

We have tried both segmentation and classification methods on this data. The segmentation of GPS paths appears in the ecology literature where two features are apparent:

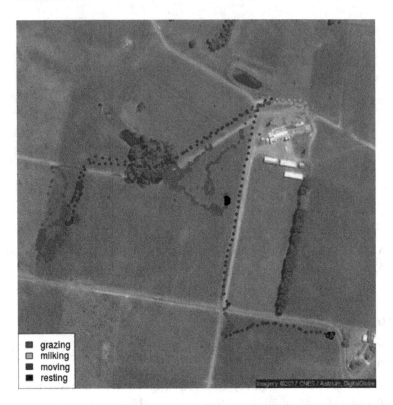

Fig. 11. A classified trajectory for Animal 6, day 2. This animal was not included in either the test or the training data. The trajectory has been cleaned up with the two heuristic rules.

- the location of the animal is interesting information in itself;
- it is likely that training data is unavailable as direct observation of the animal over an extended period may not be possible.

We have a somewhat different situation. We have some prior knowledge about the behaviour of the animals at different times and locations. We can use this knowledge to both produce and evaluate the classified trajectories. Our problem is to automate this process. Consider the following three segmentations of the same trajectory (animal 6 on day 2):

- Figure 4, the Gueguen segmentation. This has separated moving and grazing. There are occasional rest periods mixed with the grazing. However, the overall segmentation is not unreasonable;
- Figure 6, the Lavielle segmentation into 4 classes. It has separated moving from everything else but has not successfully segmented the other classes;
- Figure 11, an animal classified on 10 min segments, not included in either test or training data. The classification combined with the heuristic rules has made the trajectory quite interpretable.

The classification method appears to perform better than the segmentation methods. This may be due to the fact that is based on the 5 derived variables which give more information than the successive positions.

4 Discussion

We anticipate that the GPS data will only be able to separate the behaviour into a small number of distinct activities. Clearly, GPS information will not let us distinguish between sleeping, drowsing or ruminating. In addition the continuous small errors in GPS readings may make a stationary animal indistinguishable from a slowly moving one. This will cause some confounding of resting (Fig. 12) and grazing (Fig. 13). Both trajectories fail the Wald-Wolfowitz runs test [11] for randomness, although we suspect that only the resting (Fig. 12) trajectory is in fact random noise.

The segmentation achieved by the Gueguen method (Fig. 4) appears reasonable. It appears that the class with the smallest mean does not cover the milking. There are times in the grazing paddock when the animal is more consistently stationary than in the milking shed. However, the segmentation is relatively easy to align with our prior knowledge of the animals behavior.

The Lavielle method suggests 3 behavior classes (Fig. 5). We have selected 4 classes for an easier comparison with other methods. However the resulting segmentation (Fig. 6) make little sense.

Using the ten minute segments (Sect. 2.4) gives us a reasonable classification, shown in Fig. 9.

Table 1. Summary of the grazing behavior of Animal 6 and 29.

	Animal 6		Animal 29	
	Time (minutes)	Distance (meters)	Time (minutes)	Distance (meters)
27/11/12	676.83	4327.20	601.17	3925.46
28/11/12	892.67	4779.78	759.33	4345.09
29/11/12	908.33	4759.01	774.00	4102.31
30/11/12	796.00	4855.96	675.00	3918.92
01/12/12	820.17	4810.77	696.17	3199.86
02/12/12	857.00	3868.14	738.33	3392.88
03/12/12	836.17	5227.78	699.00	3853.94
04/12/12	839.67	5098.36	725.17	3990.13
05/12/12	847.00	5536.96	738.33	4155.51
06/12/12	857.33	5047.15	726.50	3507.63
07/12/12	885.00	4323.86	359.33	1952.70
08/12/12	242.67	783.91	250.17	1164.36
09/12/12	NA	NA	466.17	2508.31

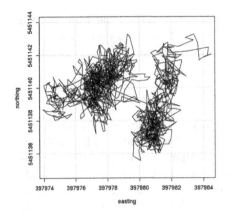
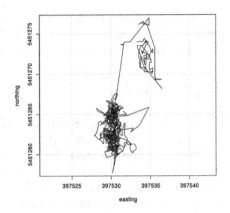

Fig. 12. Animal 6, day 2 from midnight to 04:15. We assume that the animal is resting.

Fig. 13. Animal 6, day 2 from 9:30 to 11:15, the animal is grazing

Using the method of Sect. 2.4 and two simple heuristic rules we can produce an acceptable classification of the GPS trajectory of a dairy cow into the 4 classes: milking, moving, grazing and resting. Using the classification we can produce a summary of time spent grazing and distance covered for each animal in the sample. This in given in Table 1 for animals 6 and 29.

The information derived from the classified trajectories has a number of potential uses. By itself it may indicate individual animals that are not moving well. It may also indicate some features of herd behaviour, including different spatial behaviour in different paddocks.

Its utility will increase when joined with other data (milk yield, for example) to produce a summary useful in animal management. These methods have the potential to yield important and useful information for animal management at quite a low cost.

References

1. Herd intelligence, scr. Accessed 05 Oct 2016
2. Moomonitor+ (2016). Accessed 05 Oct 2016
3. Allen, J.D., Anderson, S.D., Collier, R.J., Smith, J.F.: Managing heat stress and its impact on cow behavior. In: Proceedings of Western Dairy Management Conference, pp. 150–162 (2013)
4. Allflex. Healthycow24. Accessed 05 Oct 2016
5. Animal Behaviour. Resources for applied ethology (2016). Accessed 05 Oct 2016
6. Calenge, C.: The package adehabitat for the R software: tool for the analysis of space and habitat use by animals. Ecol. Model. **197**, 1035 (2006)

7. González, L., Schwartzkopf-Genswein, K., Caulkett, N., Janzen, E., McAllister, T., Fierheller, E., Schaefer, A., Haley, D., Stookey, J., Hendrick, S.: Pain mitigation after band castration of beef calves and its effects on performance, behavior, escherichia coli, and salivary cortisol. J. Animal Sci. **88**(2), 802–810 (2010). Cited by 38
8. Guéguen, L.: Segmentation by maximal predictive partitioning according to composition biases. In: Gascuel, O., Sagot, M.-F. (eds.) JOBIM 2000. LNCS, vol. 2066, pp. 32–44. Springer, Heidelberg (2001). doi:10.1007/3-540-45727-5_4
9. Lavielle, M.: Using penalized contrasts for the change-point problem. Signal Process. **85**(8), 1501–1510 (2005)
10. von Keyserling, M., Rushen, J., de Passille, A., Weary, D.: Behaviour of lame cows, pp. 581–588 (2011)
11. Wald, A., Wolfowitz, J.: An exact test for randomness in the non-parametric case based on serial correlation. Ann. Math. Statist. **14**(4), 378–388 (1943)
12. Wark, T., Corke, P., Sikka, P., Klingbeil, L., Guo, Y., Crossman, C., Valencia, P., Swain, D., Bishop-Hurley, G.: Transforming agriculture through pervasive wireless sensor networks. IEEE Pervasive Comput. **6**, 50–57 (2007)
13. Weary, D., Huzzey, J., Von Keyserlingk, M.: Board-invited review: using behavior to predict and identify ill health in animals. J. Animal Sci. **87**(2), 770–777 (2009)
14. Wisconsin Milk Marketing Board. Rumination or cud chewing (2016). Accessed 05 Dec 2016

Dynamic Real-Time Segmentation and Recognition of Activities Using a Multi-feature Windowing Approach

Ahmad Shahi[1]([⊠]), Brendon J. Woodford[1], and Hanhe Lin[2]

[1] Department of Information Science, University of Otago,
PO Box 56, Dunedin 9054, New Zealand
ahmad.shahi@postgrad.otago.ac.nz, brendon.woodford@otago.ac.nz
[2] Department of Computer and Information Science,
University of Konstanz, Konstanz, Germany
hanhe.lin@uni-konstanz.de

Abstract. Segmenting sensor events for activity recognition has many key challenges due to its unsupervised nature, the real-time requirements necessary for on-line event detection, and the possibility of having to recognise overlapping activities. A further challenge is to achieve robustness of classification due to sub-optimal choice of window size. In this paper, we present a novel real-time recognition framework to address these problems. The proposed framework is divided into two phases: off-line modeling and on-line recognition. In the off-line phase a representation called Activity Features (AFs) are built from statistical information about the activities from annotated sensory data and a Naïve Bayesian (NB) classifier is modeled accordingly. In the on-line phase, a dynamic multi-feature windowing approach using AFs and the learnt NB classifier is introduced to segment unlabeled sensor data as well as predicting the related activity. How this on-line segmentation occurs, even in the presence of overlapping activities, diverges from many other studies. Experimental results demonstrate that our framework can outperform the state-of-the-art windowing-based approaches for activity recognition involving datasets acquired from multiple residents in smart home test-beds.

Keywords: Human activity recognition · On-line stream mining · Real-time · Machine learning · Classification

1 Introduction

Sensor data segmentation for activity recognition is attracting increased attention at a time when greater importance is being attached to controlling, safety (e.g. health) and security in a smart home environment. However, there are a number of challenges, namely the streaming nature of the sensor data and the real-time sensor data processing requirements. As a result, most existing windowing approaches [13,14,20] that were applied in the training part or in batch

© Springer International Publishing AG 2017
U Kang et al. (Eds.): PAKDD 2017 Workshops, LNAI 10526, pp. 26–38, 2017.
DOI: 10.1007/978-3-319-67274-8_3

mode require the sensor data to have annotated labels. In the testing phase, most researchers used a fixed time or sensor-based window for segmentation [2,7,17]. An important challenge with a fixed window size is identifying the optimal window size *a priori* and as a result, many of the classification and modeling errors come from the selection of this window length [5]. Various heuristics such as the mean length of the activities and sampling frequency of the sensors were employed to determine this [9]. For example, the Sensor Window Mutual Information approach [9] is computed off-line using the training sensor sequence which then uses a fixed window size for calculating feature vectors. They also developed a method called Dynamic Window which is a probabilistic method to derive the window size automatically using a data-driven approach. However, this method still uses a fixed window sizes which correspond to the mean window size of an activity. Because of their assumption that there are no significant changes to the routine of a resident in the smart home, the window sizes for sensory data are computed using this probability in both the training and testing parts [9]. Similarly, in [12], a dynamic segmentation model was proposed where the window is shrunk and expanded based on using temporal activity information, sensor data, and the current state of activity recognition. However, this research on activity recognition did not accurately consider the segmentation of streaming unlabeled sensory data beyond the training phase. Although [1] did consider adaptation and evolution of sensory data beyond the training phase, they still used a fixed window to segment the sensor data. Dealing with an on-line stream, this model is learnt continuously, incrementally and the stream data is split into equal sized chunks only of unlabeled data [1]. Although the above approaches have achieved comparable recognition results, there is no robust solution to the problem of segmenting unlabelled streamed data. Therefore, delivering appropriately robust activity recognition systems that could be deployed with confidence in an on-line setting remains an outstanding challenge.

In this paper, we propose a novel real-time recognition framework to both segment and recognise activities using an adaptive windowing approach. Our proposed framework consists of two phases. In the off-line phase, Activity Features (AFs) are built from annotated sensory data and a Naïve Bayesian (NB) classifier is learnt subsequently. The AFs maintain the statistical information about the activities. In the on-line phase, a dynamic multi-feature windowing method using AFs is introduced to segment the unlabeled sensory data in a real-time setting. As a result, the recognition performance has been improved by the proposed framework. This framework is easy to implement, attains better results in comparison with the-state-of-the-art approaches, and recognizes overlapped activities in a real-time manner. The details of our proposed framework are described in the following section.

2   Real-Time Recognition Framework

In this section, we introduce our novel real-time recognition framework for activities along with its phases and components in a smart home environment that

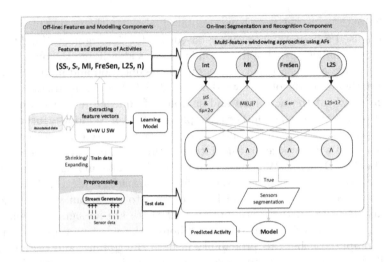

Fig. 1. Framework of activity modeling and recognition.

is depicted in Fig. 1. In terms of the windowing paradigm, the framework is divided into two phases: off-line modeling and on-line recognition. Preprocessing and modeling components are conducted in the off-line phase. In this phase, we applied an adaptive windowing model to read the sensor data based on annotated labels. An adaptive windowing method for streaming sensor data uses three elements: window length adaptation (shrinking and/or expanding the window), a time decay function, and a scheme for accommodating past sensor information.

Sensor data, S, at time, t, is read into a Sensor Window, SW, ($SW \leftarrow SW \cup S_t$). If the length of SW is less than or equal to an initial size then the activity is recognized and SW is added to the window data matrix, W. Otherwise, if Size(SW) is exhausted, the initial size will be expanded by a predefined extension value (ext), but this is expanded once only. Finally, if an activity is not recognized during reading the sensors and Size(SW) is exhausted after the expansion, the sensor data is added to the Past Sensor Information pool, which stores potentially useful information for the next window. The details of this method are elaborated in [15]. This phase is where the NB classifier and AFs are built from the annotated sensory data.

In this paper, however, our main focus and key challenge is addressing the on-line recognition phase. A dynamic multi-feature windowing approach using AFs in this phase is introduced to segment the unlabeled sensory data in a real-time setting. The details of this method is elaborated in Sect. 2.2.

2.1   Activity Features

In this study, we address Interval (Int) time, Mutual Information (MI), frequency of triggered sensors of an activity ($FreSen$) and last two sensors ($L2S$) as the features of an activity. The motivation for extracting the activity features is to carry out an activity in the recognition task. *Int* time is an effective feature to segment activities with distinct durations. *MI* shows how sensors are dependent on one another in the sequence to determine an activity. *FreSen* cares about the occurrences of activated sensors for an activity rather than the sequence of sensors. There is other information about the sensor that can aid in recognizing an activity which is called *L2S*. In a smart home test-bed, numerous activities have taken place, many sensors are triggered as the last sensor for the same activity. In other words, an activity does not carry only one sensor as a last sensor. Therefore, in this research we consider last two sensors of an activity.

Table 1. Notation of Activity Features (AFs)

Symbol	Description
MI	Mutual Information [9]
FreSen	Frequency of activated sensors in an activity [20]
L2S	Last two (2) sensors of an activity
Int	Time interval of an activity

Most scholars used a fixed time or sensor-based window for segmentation of sensor data in a real-time environment [9]. Moreover, they have not yet carefully considered on-line recognition of overlapping activities with multiple-residents. However, to tackle these aforementioned issues, we propose new approach which is called a dynamic multi-feature windowing method using Activity Features (AFs). The features and notations of AFs are described in Table 1. The AFs approach maintains the statistical information about the activities in a smart home test-bed. The information in AFs is extracted in the off-line phase which are the features (Fs) of each activity in an entire stream of training data. These features of activities are defined as temporal feature vectors. The properties of AFs assist the sensors stream to be recognized in an on-line fashion. The details of AFs are elaborated as follows.

Sensor Dependency Using Mutual Information. "Mutual Information" (*MI*) [9] measures how much one random variable tells us about another. The *MI* or dependence between two sensors is then defined as the chance that these two sensors occur consecutively in the entire sensor stream. More formally, if S_i and S_j are two sensors, then the $MI(i,j)$ between them is defined as

$$MI(i,j) = \frac{1}{N} \sum_{K=1}^{N-1} \delta(S_k, S_i)\delta(S_{k+1}, S_j) \tag{1}$$

where $\delta(S_k, S_i)$ takes value of 1 if $S_k = S_i$ and 0 otherwise. S_j is a subsequent of S_i, the summation term takes value 1 otherwise it takes the value of 0, and N is the number of activated sensors in an activity.

Frequency of Activated Sensors for an Activity. In MI, the sequence of the sensors are considered within an entire stream while sometimes an activity behaves with a different order of sensor events. In addition, some sensors do not necessary happen in order, however are still part of an activity. The example presents the idea clearly which is as follows. **(1)** $A_1{:}S_1 \to S_2 \to S_3 \to S_1 \to S_2 \to S_4$, **(2)** $A_1{:}S_1 \to S_3 \to S_2 \to S_1 \to S_4 \to S_2$. Assuming that the first path is statistically less used than the second path but both paths lead to the same activity, we can clearly see that there is a dependency between sensors S_1 and S_2 whichever path is used. If we adopt the previous way for computing the MI between sensors S_1 and S_2, we will lose some dependency information between them. Furthermore, there are activities that are often performed in parallel, and sensor events of an activity can be descriptive for the other and MI cannot take this situation into account.

Based on these assumptions, $FreSen$ method was proposed in [20] to compute the probability between two sensors S_i and S_j by calculating their frequency of occurrence in the space of N sensor events for an activity along the entire training data stream, as defined by the following equations:

$$FreSen^i(k,j) = \frac{1}{N} \sum_{l=1}^{N} \delta_f(S_k, S_j) \tag{2}$$

$$\delta_f(S_k, S_j) = \begin{cases} 1 & \text{if } \{S_k, S_j\} \in E_i \\ 0 & \text{otherwise} \end{cases} \tag{3}$$

where N is the number of activated sensors in an activity, $\delta_f(S_k, S_j)$ takes value of 1 if S_k and S_j activated in E_i where E_i stands for sensor events in activity, A_i, and 0 otherwise. $FreSen$ as an activity feature vector in an entire stream, is a list of activated sensors for each activity. Therefore, inspired by the $FreSen$ which is described in Definition 1, the acceptable sensors for an activity are those having a high probability of occurring. This candidate selection is first set of maximum probabilities such that their summation is less than and equal to 95%. The definition below describes the histogram of frequency of activated sensors for an activity.

Definition 1. For each S_{ij} in an activity (A_i), $S_{ij} = \{\forall S_j \in A_i | j = 1, \ldots, N, i = 1, \ldots, M\}$, the sensors with the highest probabilities are considered as the first set of candidates for selection that is shown in Eq. (4). Let P_{ij} is a probability of S_j in A_i (all sensors in P_i are sorted in descending order). Thus, the list of activated sensors with high probability for activity A_i is:

$$P^i_{final}(S) = \{S | \text{argmax} \sum_{j=1}^{N} \{P_{ij} | P^i_{final}(S_j) \le 0.95|\}\} \tag{4}$$

In other words, the occurrences of sensors in a reading of them for an activity A_i, should not exceed the error threshold, T, which is set at 0.05:

$$err = a + \frac{(b-a)(w_j - P_{min})}{P_{max} - P_{min}} \tag{5}$$

$$w_j = \log \frac{1}{P_j + \lambda} \qquad (6)$$

where, $[P_{min}, P_{max}] \leftarrow [0, \log(\frac{1}{\lambda}) + 1]$ and $[a, b] \leftarrow [0, T]$. In Eq. (6) the weight, w, of a sensor is computed based on the probability of a sensor that happened for an activity. However, some sensors might not have occurred for an activity. Therefore, the probability of the sensor would be zero which means w would lead to infinity without adding some type of offset. To avoid infinity, we applied a Laplace correction to the estimate of w_j by adding a small value, $\lambda > 0$, to the probability of the sensor as shown in Eq. (6). After computing the weight of occurrences of sensor in an activity, we normalized the weights in a predefined period $[a, b]$ that is depicted in Eq. (5).

Last Two-State Sensor Method. For an activity, several sensor events might be triggered and sometimes the last sensor event of an activity is more descriptive than the previous sensors [9]. However, by an increment in the number of activities or sensors the chance of overlap, synchronization or swapping in triggering sensors grows. To overcome this drawback, i.e. last two sensors alternation, we merge last two sensors and consider them as a whole. In another word, in our research, we consider last two sensors as a "last sensor". This is because we believe that sometimes the last two sensors of an activity are much more descriptive when they occasionally activate before or after each other. As intimated earlier, a resident can take the path in both ways (1 and 2) for the same activity A_1. For path 1, the last and second last sensors are S_4 and S_2 respectively. While for the path 2 the last and second last sensors are S_2 and S_4 respectively. The reason for considering the last two sensors of an activity is that a resident may switch the activation of these last two sensors for the same activity.

Therefore, in constructing AFs, one of the conditions for feature extraction and segmentation is considering the last two sensors (S_{i-1}, S_i). S_i and S_{i-1} are assumed to be last and second last sensors respectively. During segmentation when S_i is checked as last sensor, S_{i-1} is taken as an extra feature for subsequent on-line segmentation to be checked whether it is activated as its previous sensor or not. If not, as mentioned earlier, the two sensors might be triggered before or after the other. Therefore, (S_i, S_{i-1}) is considered either is the last two events in an activity segmentation or not. The mathematical representation of last two sensors $(L2S)$ is depicted in Eqs. (7)–(9):

$$L2S(S_k, S_i) = \log_2 \left(\frac{f(S_k, S_i) + g(S_k, S_i)}{f(S_k, S_i)g(S_k, S_i) + 1} + 1 \right) \qquad (7)$$

$$f(S_k, S_i) = \delta(S_k, S_i)\delta(S_{k-1}, S_{i-1}) \qquad (8)$$

$$g(S_k, S_i) = \delta(S_k, S_{i-1})\delta(S_{k-1}, S_i) \qquad (9)$$

where $\delta(S_k, S_i)$ takes value of 1 if $S_k = S_i$ and 0 otherwise. S_i is assumed to be the last sensor and S_k is a sensor which is read from the data stream. Thus, Eq. (8) checks whether S_k is the last sensor or not. If so, it also checks its previous sensor (S_{k-1}) that should be the second last sensor $(S_{k-1} = S_{i-1})$. As previously stated, the last two sensors sometimes appear before or after the other. Thus, Eq. (9) checks S_i as a last sensor that might appear as a second last sensor $(S_{k-1} = S_i)$. Besides, its previous sensor (S_{i-1}) might behave as if is the last sensor $(S_k = S_{i-1})$ which is still valid for S_i to be considered as the last sensor. Equation (7) then returns 0 or 1 for checking the last two sensors. If $L2S = 0$ means the sensor S_k and S_i are not the last two sensors. On the other hand, If $L2S = 1$ means the sensor S_k and S_i are the last two sensors.

Activity Time Interval. As mentioned in AFs, one of the features for segmentation is the time interval, Int, of an activity in an on-line stream. In a time interval, the sum of the squares of the time stamp sensor, SS_T, and sum of a set of time-stamp sensors (S_T) of an activity, A_i, are formulated in Eqs. (10) and (11) respectively.

$$SS_T^i = \sum_{j=1}^{N} (T_{ij})^2 \tag{10}$$

$$S_T^i = \sum_{j=1}^{N} (T_{ij}) \tag{11}$$

where T_{ij} is a time stamp of an activated sensor S_j for an activity A_i and N is a number of activated sensors for activity A_i which is varied for each activity. We note that the time stamp data allows us to calculate the mean and standard deviation[1] of the time interval of activities in a given AFs. The windowing of reading sensors for an activity based on AFs should satisfy the mean interval and should not exceed $(\mu + 2\sigma)$, where μ is the mean and σ is the standard deviation.

2.2   Dynamic Multi-feature Windowing Approach

Each AF alone is capable of contributing to classifying sensor data. However, to achieve more accurate segmentation as well as recognition, we proposed a multi-feature windowing approach which is derived from AFs on-line to dynamically

Table 2. Notation of dynamic multi-feature windowing approaches for segmentation.

Notation	Description
MI_Int	Combining AFs of MI and Int
MI_FreSen_Int	Combining AFs of MI, $FreSen$, and Int
MI_L2S_Int	Combining AFs of MI, $L2S$, and Int
$FreSen\_L2S\_Int$	Combining AFs of $FreSen$, $L2S$, and Int

---

[1] The   mean   is   equal   to S_T/N.   The   standard   deviation   is   equal   to $\sqrt{(SS_T/N) - (S_T/N)^2}$.

segment unlabeled streamed data. For the windowing purposes, we considered using multi-feature of AFs to segment sensor data precisely which is described in Table 2. The *Int* feature is an essential and meaningful feature of AFs that holds the time-stamp for an activity. The *L2S* feature is a flag that maintains extra information to assist other features to segment unlabeled sensor data. Our modified *FreSen* holds important information about a sensor of activities as well as providing a threshold for segmentation. For instance, the *FreSen_L2S_Int* approach is used to segment the streaming sensory data by meeting the conditions of *FreSen* with high probability, *L2S*, and *Int* in a segment. Algorithm 1 details the multi-feature method using AFs.

Multi-feature windowing approaches combine more features to segment the sensor data in an on-line fashion. Indeed, multi-feature methods are appealing mainly because they are able to improve on a single feature which can make more accurate recognition. On the other hand, in a smart home test-bed, different activities trigger a similar set of sensors which causes overlapping activities. Nevertheless, our proposed dynamic multi-feature method is able to distinguish these overlapping activities. A clear example of overlapping is depicted in Fig. 2. When sensors are triggered, our multi-feature method reads unlabeled sensor data and segments them based on the generated AFs. These sensors are added to all available activities windows until meeting the condition criteria (the condition of features are checked using the CheckConditions() function as shown in

---

Algorithm 1. Multi-feature windowing approach

Require: $MI \leftarrow$ Prior probability $P^i(S_{j-1}, S_j)$ of sequence sensors for activity A_i; $FreSen \leftarrow$ Sort the prior probability (P_S^i) of sensors for activity A_i where $i = 1, \ldots, m$ in descending order $(list[P_S^i])$;
$L2S_i \leftarrow list\{S_{j-1}, S_j\}^i$ where $j = 1, \ldots, N$; $Int \leftarrow [\mu, \sigma]$ for each activity;
$W_i \leftarrow S_1$ Initial window of activities with first activated sensor;
Define: Multi-feature functions $\{f_c, c = 1, \ldots, C\}$

while *active* **do**
    $S_j \leftarrow$ getNextSensor(); // Read arriving stream data.
    for $i \leftarrow 1$ *to* m **do**
        $W_i \leftarrow W_i \cup S_j$;
        foreach c *in* C **do**
            $status =$ CheckConditions(f_c^i, S_j);
        // $status = true$ means the conditions were satisfied.
        if $status == true$ **then**
            extractFeatureVector(W_i); // Segment the window and pass for extracting features vector.
            $W_i =$ Recreate(W_i); // Discard and create new window of W_i.
        else
            // $status = false$, then discard and create new window of W_i.
            $W_i =$ Recreate(W_i);

Algorithm 1) and is elaborated in Subsect. 2.1 for each feature). If a window did not satisfy the all conditions of the features for an activity, the window is discarded and a new activity window is created for reading activated sensor events. Figure 2 which is a graphical presentation of Algorithm 1, shows how activities, particularly overlapping activities, are segmented. In Fig. 2, sensors S_1, S_2 and S_3 are added to segment 1 of both *Activity 1* and *Activity 2*. However, *Activity 2* did not satisfy the conditions and has been discarded. Right after, a new window of *Activity 2* is created to read incoming activated sensors S_2 and S_4. The same procedure is performed for Segment 2 of *Activity 2* which is overlapping with Segment 2 of *Activity 1*.

2.3   Our Machine Learning Technique for Activity Recognition

In this paper, we use a NB classifier as a learner with Bernoulli distribution [8] for modeling streaming sensory data in real-time applications. Because the learning algorithm is very simple, efficient, effective, and it is therefore suitable for learning from high-speed and massive data streams [11]. NB classifier whose posteriori probability computed by $P(y_i|x) = \frac{P(x|y_i)P(y_i)}{P(x)}$, where $0 < p < 1$; x is one with binary outcomes which $\in \{0,1\}$; $P(y_i)$: prior; $P(x|y_i) = \prod_j p_j^{x_j}(1-p_j)^{1-x_j}$: conditional probability modeled based on Bernoulli probabilities of sensor values. For each classifier, classification decision made based on Maximum Likelihood Posteriori $\phi_k(x) = \underset{i}{\mathrm{argmax}}\, P(y_i|x)$.

Handling Binary Attributes and Laplace Correction. To model the binary Bernoulli distribution for sensor events, the amount of training data might not be sufficient and the value v_j of binary attribute x_j may not be observed in class y_i. So, $P(x_j = v_j|y_i) = 0$, causing $P(y_i|x)$ to become zero. Hence, it is necessary to employ the Laplace correction to the estimate of $P(x_j = v_{js}|y_i)$ by adding

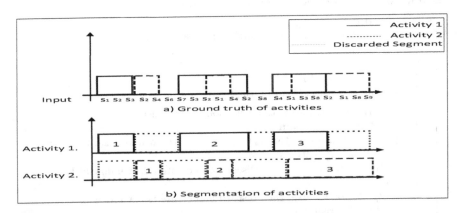

Fig. 2. An example of segmenting overlapped activities using dynamic multi-feature method using AFs.

a small offset, $\lambda > 0$, to the frequency n_{ij}: $P(x_j = v_{js}|y_i) = \frac{n_{ijs}+\lambda}{n_i+m_j\lambda}$, where $m_j = 2$: the number of values for attribute x_j and $\lambda = 1$ as referred to in [11].

3 Experimental Results

To evaluate our proposed approach, we used real-world datasets from the Washington State University (WSU) CASAS smart home project. We chose three datasets: Tulum 2009 [4], Tulum 2009/2010 and Aruba [3].

3.1 Evaluation Metrics

To evaluate the performance of our proposed methods in a real-time setting, we split the data into training (80% of the data) and testing (20% of the data) parts [19] where the training data used off-line to build the learning model and AFs. The remaining unlabeled stream data is applied for testing the methods and labels are only revealed for the evaluation purposes. For the measurement, we used accuracy, F-score and sequence alignment score metrics as detailed below:

A. Accuracy: Let N_{A_i} be the total number of sensor windows associated with a predefined activity A_i and the number of correctly classified windows for this predefined activity be TP_{A_i}. The activity classification accuracy can then be defined as: $\sum_{i=1}^{m} \frac{TP_{A_i}}{N_{A_i}}$, where m is the total number of predefined activities.

B. F-score: Let P and R represent the precision and recall for activity A_i, then the F-score for this activity is computed as: $2 \times \frac{P \times R}{P+R}$. As an overall metric, accuracy is not sufficient to evaluate the classifier performance [6,16], because the minority classes will be dominated by majority classes. However, the F-score is included as an appropriate metric; particularly for having imbalanced data.

C. Sequence Alignment Score: We use the Sequence Alignment-Needleman Wunsch Algorithm [10] to evaluate methods in a sequential manner. In this algorithm, the maximum match is a number dependent upon the similarity of the sequences. The details are elaborated in [10]. As an example, let us define two sequences, B and D, as follows: B: $A_4A_2A_2A_1A_1A_4A_2$, D: $A_4A_3A_3A_1A_2A_4A_1A_2$. Therefore, an alignment of B and D will be where $\{\forall b \in B, \forall d \in D\}$, *Match:* $+8$ $\{F(b,d) = 8|b = d)\}$, *Mismatch:* -2 $\{F(b,d) = -2|b <> d)\}$, and each *gap symbol:* -2 $\{F(b,d) = -2|b = \text{'-'} \vee d = \text{'-'}\}$. Thus, the alignment score will be 20.

3.2 Results and Analyses

We have carried out experiments on three data sets (as illustrated in Sect. 3) using the baseline and proposed multi-feature windowing methods. These methods and their notations are summarized for clarity in Table 2. The performance of the state-of-the-art and multi-feature windowing methods for reading sensor data stream in activities recognition in a real-time environment are shown in Table 3.

Table 3. Evaluation of multi-feature approaches using AFs.

Metrics/Methods	MI	FreSen	MI_Int	MI_FreSen_Int	MI_L2S_Int	FreSen_L2S_Int
Tulum2009						
Accuracy (%)	4.76	15.3	**87.5**	80	80	63.63
F-score	0.6909	0.7142	**0.9538**	0.9333	0.9387	0.8235
Alignment score	−33884	−226	−4486	−82	−138	42
Tulum2010						
Accuracy (%)	65.71	48	**91.42**	84	90.74	84.21
F-score	0.8051	0.6581	0.9241	0.9124	**0.9435**	0.8974
Alignment score	−1952	14	−960	−4	12	**20**
Aruba						
Accuracy (%)	75.30	65.79	94.28	**100**	80.74	**100**
F-score	0.8533	0.8758	0.9565	**1**	0.8069	**1**
Alignment score	−2378	−1002	−960	**14**	−40	4

As shown in this table we evaluated the performance of baseline methods namely *MI* and *FreSen*. [9] argued that *MI* outperforms the fixed time and sensor-based windows. On the other hand, [18] proved the *FreSen* method gives better presentation and precise results compared to *MI*. However, these methods did not segment the unlabeled sensor data in a real-time environment. Thus, our multi-feature windowing methods could even segment this data with overlapping activities. Table 3 also demonstrates that *MI_FreSen_Int* features allows the NB classifier to achieve 100% accuracy on Aruba dataset whereas the combination *MI_Int* features obtained much better performance on Tulum2009 and Tulum2010 datasets. On the other hand, the accuracy of using only *MI* or *FreSen* features on Tulum2009 dataset is very low. This is because of the level of imbalance between classes within these different datasets. Thus, the accuracy is not a proper metric to evaluate the classier performance. Overall, our proposed approaches against the *MI* and *FreSen* methods attained comparable or better results with regard to accuracy, F-score, and alignment score metrics which are shown in Table 3.

It is worth mentioning that the performance of fixed-time and sensor-based windows is poor when the length of the window is static for reading sensor events [9]. While, our proposed multi-feature windowing approach has the advantage of giving more confidence as well as providing more information for the segmentation. Thus, we suggest that performance in adopting multi-features is better over the use of a single feature. The experiments showed that the performance of our proposed methods is better than the baseline methods in a real-time setting.

3.3 Run-Time Analysis

The approaches are implemented using the C# .NET programming language and run on a computer using Windows 7 Professional (64-bit operating system)

Table 4. Average running-time of approaches on Tulum2009, Tulum2010 and Aruba datasets in a real-time setting (milliseconds/segment).

Datasets/methods	MI	$FreSen$	MI_Int	MI_FreSen_Int	MI_L2S_Int	$FreSen\_L2S\_Int$
Tulum2009	1.77	15.73	0.6251	1.34	1.22	2.64
Tulum2010	3.22	6.45	3.2	7.24	10.75	26.93
Aruba	1.75	15.54	1.83	20.17	4.23	151.41

with an Intel Quad Core i5 CPU @ 3.40 GHz and 8 GB of memory. Table 4 shows the average running-time of the methods in milliseconds (ms) per segment. The running-time of some methods (e.g. *FreSen_L2S_Int*) are higher. The main reason is that, some activities (e.g. *Sleeping and Watching TV*) have a longer duration. Therefore, segmenting such activities also takes longer. For instance, when testing the Aruba dataset, most activities are *Sleeping* or *Watching TV*.

4 Conclusion

Segmenting unlabeled streaming sensor data from smart home test-beds is a challenging task especially when there is a need to recognize overlapping events due to multiple residents inhabiting the house. In this paper we presented a novel recognition framework to address these problems by using the AFs to dynamically segment this data in combination with a NB classifier to recognize such activities even when they are overlapping. Experimental results demonstrated that our approach achieved better results compared with state-of-the-art windowing approaches. In the future, we intend to focus on modeling activities in order to find abnormal behaviors using a probabilistic graphical model in a real-time setting.

References

1. Abdallah, Z.S., Gaber, M.M., Srinivasan, B., Krishnaswamy, S.: Adaptive mobile activity recognition system with evolving data streams. Neurocomputing **150**, 304–317 (2015)
2. Bao, L., Intille, S.S.: Activity recognition from user-annotated acceleration data. In: Ferscha, A., Mattern, F. (eds.) Pervasive 2004. LNCS, vol. 3001, pp. 1–17. Springer, Heidelberg (2004). doi:10.1007/978-3-540-24646-6_1
3. Cook, D.J.: Learning setting-generalized activity models for smart spaces. IEEE Intell. Syst. **27**(1), 32–38 (2012)
4. Cook, D.J., Schmitter-Edgecombe, M.: Assessing the quality of activities in a smart environment. Methods Inf. Med. **48**(5), 480–485 (2009)
5. Gu, T., Wu, Z., Tao, X., Pung, H.K., Lu, J.: epsicar: an emerging patterns based approach to sequential, interleaved and concurrent activity recognition. In: IEEE International Conference on Pervasive Computing and Communications (PerCom 2009), pp. 1–9. IEEE (2009)

6. He, H., Garcia, E.A.: Learning from imbalanced data. IEEE Trans. Knowl. Data Eng. **21**(9), 1263–1284 (2009)
7. Huỳnh, T., Blanke, U., Schiele, B.: Scalable recognition of daily activities with wearable sensors. In: Hightower, J., Schiele, B., Strang, T. (eds.) LoCA 2007. LNCS, vol. 4718, pp. 50–67. Springer, Heidelberg (2007). doi:10.1007/978-3-540-75160-1_4
8. Johnson, N.L., Kemp, A.W., Kotz, S.: Univariate Discrete Distributions, vol. 444. Wiley, Hoboken (2005)
9. Krishnan, N.C., Cook, D.J.: Activity recognition on streaming sensor data. Pervasive Mob. Comput. **10**, 138–154 (2014)
10. Needleman, S.B., Wunsch, C.D.: A general method applicable to the search for similarities in the amino acid sequence of two proteins. J. Mol. Biol. **48**(3), 443–453 (1970)
11. Nguyen, H.M., Cooper, E.W., Kamei, K.: Online learning from imbalanced data streams. In: 2011 International Conference of Soft Computing and Pattern Recognition (SoCPaR), pp. 347–352. IEEE (2011)
12. Okeyo, G., Chen, L., Wang, H., Sterritt, R.: Dynamic sensor data segmentation for real-time knowledge-driven activity recognition. Pervasive Mob. Comput. **10**, 155–172 (2014)
13. Peterek, T., Penhaker, M., Gajdoš, P., Dohnálek, P.: Comparison of classification algorithms for physical activity recognition. In: Abraham, A., Krömer, P., Snášel, V. (eds.) Innovations in Bio-inspired Computing and Applications. Advances in Intelligent Systems and Computing, vol. 237, pp. 123–131. Springer, Cham (2014). doi:10.1007/978-3-319-01781-5_12
14. Preece, S.J., Goulermas, J.Y., Kenney, L.P., Howard, D., Meijer, K., Crompton, R.: Activity identification using body-mounted sensorsa review of classification techniques. Physiol. Meas. **30**(4), R1–R33 (2009)
15. Shahi, A., Woodford, B.J., Deng, J.D.: Event classification using adaptive cluster-based ensemble learning of streaming sensor data. In: Pfahringer, B., Renz, J. (eds.) AI 2015. LNCS, vol. 9457, pp. 505–516. Springer, Cham (2015). doi:10.1007/978-3-319-26350-2_45
16. Sobhani, P., Viktor, H., Matwin, S.: Learning from imbalanced data using ensemble methods and cluster-based undersampling. In: Appice, A., Ceci, M., Loglisci, C., Manco, G., Masciari, E., Ras, Z.W. (eds.) NFMCP 2014. LNCS, vol. 8983, pp. 69–83. Springer, Cham (2015). doi:10.1007/978-3-319-17876-9_5
17. Van Kasteren, T., Noulas, A., Englebienne, G., Kröse, B.: Accurate activity recognition in a home setting. In: Proceedings of the 10th International Conference on Ubiquitous Computing, pp. 1–9. ACM (2008)
18. Wan, J., O'Grady, M.J., O'Hare, G.M.: Dynamic sensor event segmentation for real-time activity recognition in a smart home context. Personal Ubiquitous Comput. **19**(2), 287–301 (2015)
19. Wiss, S., Kulikowsk, C.: Computer systems that learn: classification and prediction methods from statistics. In: Neural Networks, Machine Learning and Expert Systems. Morgan Kaufmann, San Mateo (1991)
20. Yala, N., Fergani, B., Fleury, A.: Feature extraction for human activity recognition on streaming data. In: 2015 International Symposium on Innovations in Intelligent SysTems and Applications (INISTA), pp. 1–6. IEEE (2015)

Feature Extraction from EEG Data for a P300 Based Brain-Computer Interface

Ali Hajian[✉] and Suet-Peng Yong

Universiti Teknologi PETRONAS, Seri Iskandar, Malaysia
{ali_18393,yongsuetpeng}@utp.edu.my

Abstract. Brain-computer interface (BCI) is an input method that helps users to control a computer system using their brain activity rather than a physical activity that is required when using a keyboard or mouse. BCI can be especially helpful for users with limb disabilities or limitations as it does not require any muscle movement and instead relies on user's brain activity. These brain activities are recorded using electroencephalogram (EEG). Classification of the EEG data will help to map the relevant data to certain stimuli effect. The work in this paper is aiming to find a feature extraction technique that can lead to improve the classification accuracy of EEG based BCI systems that are specifically designed for incapacitated subjects. Through the experiments, the implementation of Independent Component Analysis (ICA) and Common Spatial Pattern (CSP) extracted features from P300 based BCI EEG data and it was found that ICA and CSP produce more discriminative feature sets as compared to raw EEG signals.

Keywords: Electroencephalogram · Brain-computer interface · P300 · Independent Component Analysis · Common Spatial Pattern · Feature extraction

1 Introduction

The primary objective of BCI research is to create frameworks that enable incapacitated subjects to control their surroundings, mechanical appendages, communicate with people or command electronic devices [1]. This can be particularly helpful for incapacitated subjects in order to help them with their daily tasks. Multiple aspects of BCI systems have been investigated in order to attain this objective. Creation, assessment and validation of BCI systems that are particularly designed to be used by incapacitated subjects, creating new BCI oriented products, assessment of different brain signal measurement technologies, producing algorithms that extract computer commands from brain signals and assessment of brain signal patterns that can potentially be helpful to achieve communication (i.e. control signals) are some of these research areas [1–3].

P300 is the name of a particular human EEG positive deflection that is caused by a sudden, unexpected or shocking stimulus. It occurs about 300 ms after the

© Springer International Publishing AG 2017
U Kang et al. (Eds.): PAKDD 2017 Workshops, LNAI 10526, pp. 39–50, 2017.
DOI: 10.1007/978-3-319-67274-8_4

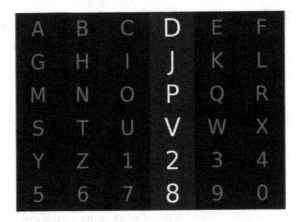

Fig. 1. Example of a P300 speller system

stimulus [4]. P300 was first used as a BCI control signal in the P300 speller system [5]. This system enables users to spell words for the computer. The user would need to choose letters sequentially from a provided table of alphabet and symbols that is presented on a computer display (Fig. 1). While columns and rows of the table are being flashed in a random and unpredictable sequence, the user would need to count the number of flashes that occur for a particular desired symbol. A P300 signal would be recorded in a user's EEG only after either the column or the row of that desired symbol is flashed. Hence it is expected that a simple algorithm would be able to detect the targeted symbol by finding the column and row that would evoke P300.

In this paper, the effect of two different feature extraction methods in a P300 based BCI system specifically designed for incapacitated subjects was investigated. The main objective of this work is to improve the classification accuracy of P300 based BCI systems. Our hypothesis is that the implementation of Independent Component Analysis (ICA) and Common Spatial Pattern (CSP) would result in a better feature set than those of raw EEG and hence an improvement in final classification accuracy.

2   Related Work

While the P300 based BCI was designed to serve the needs of incapacitated subjects, no subject who participated in the initial demonstration was disabled [5]. However, in a later work a P300 based four-choice paradigm was tested on a group of six subjects. Amongst which three subjects were suffering from a neurological disease, namely Amyotrophic Lateral Sclerosis (ALS)[1] [6]. This particular research proved that subjects suffering from ALS would be able to use P300 based BCI to ease their communication. Moreover, in a more recent

---

[1] ALS is the name of a disease that cause a loss of control over voluntary muscles.

work, using a group of nine subjects, five of which were disabled, a six-choice
P300 paradigm was evaluated. Six images were presented on a Laptop display
in front of each subject. Subjects were instructed to count the number of flashes
that occur for a prescribed targeted image. Every 400 ms, one of the images
was flashed in a random sequence and subject's EEG was recorded from 32
electrodes. Next, single trials were extracted from the recorded data by applying
a preprocessing procedure. Then, classifiers were learned using Bayesian Linear
Discriminant Analysis (BLDA) and an average classification accuracy for each
subject was estimated using four-fold cross validation. It was demonstrated that
for both normal and incapacitated subjects, a P300 based BCI can achieve a
very high accuracy rate after only a few repetitions of stimuli [1].

However, none of the works mentioned above has applied feature extraction
method to the raw EEG; the data from each electrode was simply used as one
input feature for the learning algorithm. This inspired the present work to explore
different feature extraction methods that can potentially improve the accuracy
result of the algorithm introduced in [1].

There are several feature extraction methods that are prominent when it
comes to feature learning from EEG data. ICA and CSP are two of commonly
used feature extraction methods in the preprocessing of EEG data. However,
they do not seem to be used for P300 based BCI applications [7,8].

CSP is a mathematical method that has been used in signal processing in
order to split a multivariate signal into its additive components. CSP maximizes
the difference between the variances of two classes. One of the earliest suggestions
to use CSP as a feature extraction method for EEG was given in [9]. The primary
goal of CSP is to transform EEG data into a lower dimensional space and this
linear transformation is performed using a projection matrix.

ICA is another mathematical method that extracts additive signals from a
multivariate signal [10,11]. ICA's primary assumption is that all components are
non-Gaussian (i.e. not normalized) signals and they are statistically independent
from one another. ICA can be considered a special type of a blind source separation. The most commonly known example application of ICA is the "cocktail
party problem". This problem is about the ability to concentrate on one particular stimulus while other stimuli are being filtered. Independent components
that are linearly mixed in several sensors could easily be separated using ICA.
Hence, assuming that the artefacts in EEG are commonly independent from one
another, it could be feasible for ICA to separate out artefacts from the data.

3   Methodology

The initial program and the entire dataset used in this work is based on the
work that was carried out by Hoffmann et al. at École Polytechnique Fédérale
de Lausanne (EPFL) [1].

After functionality verification, each feature extraction technique was separately applied to the dataset used in [1]. This resulted in three different versions
of the program: the original work that uses raw EEG and two modified versions

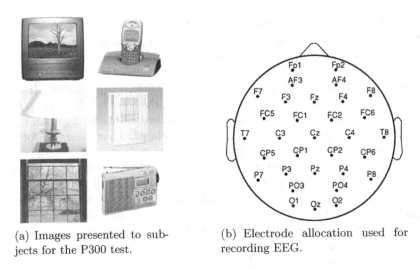

(a) Images presented to subjects for the P300 test.

(b) Electrode allocation used for recording EEG.

Fig. 2. Images and electrode allocation used in [1].

of it, one for each feature extraction method's implementation. Each version was then applied to the data separately. The result was three different sets of features selected or extracted from the same EEG dataset.

The features resulting from all three different preprocessing approaches were used to learn three separate sets of classifiers using BLDA. For each program version, a four-fold cross validation technique was used in order to estimate the classifier accuracy of that particular preprocessing approach. The accuracy results of all program versions were then compared in order to discover the preprocessing procedure that resulted in the best features among the three.

3.1 Experimental Data

Using a group of nine subjects, five of which were disabled, a six-choice of P300 paradigm was evaluated. Six images, as shown in Fig. 2, were presented on a Laptop display in front of each subject. Subjects were instructed to count the number of flashes that occur for a prescribed targeted image. Every 400 ms, one of the images was flashed in a random sequence and subject's EEG was recorded from 32 electrodes. Each flash lasted for 100 ms and no flash occurred during the 300 ms following that, this results in 400 ms of inter-stimulus interval (ISI). The data from 32 EEG electrodes was recorded with the sampling rate of 2048 Hz. 10–20 international system's standard positions were used for the placement of electrodes (Fig. 2(b)).

There were four recording sessions done by each subject. Each recording session included six runs, one for each image on the screen. Before each run, subjects were instructed to count the number of flashes that occur for a prescribed targeted image. EEG was recorded while the images were flashing in a block-randomized manner to ensure the total number of flashes for an image in each run would be equal across all images. Hence in every six consequent flashes, each image would only flash once. The total number of blocks in each run was randomly selected from the close interval of 20 to 25. This would result in an average of 22.5, 135 and 540 P300 (target) trials for each run, session and subject respectively. Moreover, for each subject a total of 3240 trials was recorded.

This resulted in a two dimensional matrix $X \in \mathbb{R}^{n \times m}$ of raw EEG recordings for each run, where n is the number of electrodes and m is the number of samples in that run.

3.2   Data Processing

In this work, there were two major data processing steps, preprocessing and classification. First, single trials were extracted from the recorded data by applying a preprocessing procedure, then classifiers were learned using BLDA and tested through a four-fold cross validation.

3.2.1   Preprocessing

The first step in processing raw EEG data is preprocessing. It needs to take place before any classification training, testing or validation is done. The detailed steps of preprocessing done in the present work in chronological order comes below:

a. Referencing: Referenced using the average of two mastoid electrodes' signals.
b. Filtering: Bandpass filter of 1.0 Hz to 12.0 Hz was applied using a sixth order forward-backward Butterworth.
c. Down sampling: Down sampling to 32 Hz took place.
d. Single trial extraction: The single trial of each stimuli begins at its start time and ends 1000 ms after that which leads to 600 ms of overlapping in every two consequent single trials.
e. Winsorizing: The data from each electrode was separately winsorized in order to decrease the influence of statistical outliers. A 10% winsorization was done using the 5th and 95th percentiles as the minimum and maximum amplitude values respectively. Any sample value greater than maximum or less than minimum was replaced by the maximum or minimum value itself.
f. Normalization[2]: Statistical normalization was applied on the data from each electrode.
g. Feature vector construction: At this step the program is divided into three different versions, the original work and two modified versions of it, one for each feature extraction method. In the original work, a group of electrodes were simply selected and no further process of data was done prior to classification. On the other hand, the present work has employed a couple of feature extraction techniques, ICA and CSP in order to construct two different sets of feature vectors.

---

[2] This step is not performed for ICA algorithm as it eliminates non-Gaussian characteristics of the data and ICA requires data to be non-Gaussian.

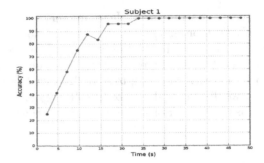

Fig. 3. Average classification accuracy over all runs for one subject. The accuracy would increase after every new block of data.

3.2.2 Classification

For each one of the three feature vectors constructed in the data preprocessing step, separate classifiers were learned using BLDA algorithm. Average classification accuracy for each subject was estimated using four-fold cross validation. The data from three sessions was used to train the classifiers. The classifiers were then validated using the data from the other session. During validation, the first 120 trials (20 blocks) were extracted from each run that is included in the validation session. 120 extracted single trials were than classified in order to produce 120 classifier outputs which means 20 blocks of six output, one output per image per block. The total classifier output for each image is calculated by adding its output values across all blocks. The image with maximum total classifier output value across all blocks would be considered the one that the subject is concentrating on. In order to simulate the time needed to achieve an average classification accuracy, the classification was done progressively for each block. This resulted in an average accuracy over all twenty-four runs for each subject as shown in Fig. 3.

3.3 Feature Extraction

As mentioned earlier, we have constructed three different sets of features using different preprocessing approaches: the original work's, the ICA's and the CSP's feature sets. By using any one of these, a different set of average accuracy results was generated for each subject. This means three sets of average accuracy results for each subject. Using all three results of all subjects, we can produce a comprehensive comparison between the three preprocessing methods and discover the one that generates features that lead us to a more accurate classifier for the present data. In this work, all results are graphed together in order to produce a cleaner comparison and help us conclude the best preprocessing method amongst the three purposed. CSP and ICA explanation follows.

3.3.1   Common Spatial Pattern

As described in [12], details of CSP algorithm using the example of EEG with target (P300) and non-target (non-P300) trials is explained as follow: X_1 and X_0 are the matrices of preprocessed EEG for target and non-target classes respectively where $X_j \in \mathrm{IR}^{N \times T \times M_j}$, N is the number of channels (electrodes), T is the number of samples per single trial (sampling rate $\times$ single trial time) and M_j is the number of single trials in the class j. Hence $X_j^i \in \mathrm{IR}^{N \times T}$ denotes a two dimensional matrix of ith single trial in X_j where $1 \leq i \leq M_j$. The normalized spatial covariance of EEG can be calculated as

$$R_1 = \Sigma_{i=1}^M \frac{X_1^i (X_1^i)^T}{trace(X_1^i (X_1^i)^T)} \tag{1}$$

and

$$R_0 = \Sigma_{i=1}^M \frac{X_0^i (X_0^i)^T}{trace(X_0^i (X_0^i)^T)} \tag{2}$$

where the normalized covariance, R_1 and R_0, are calculated by adding over covariance of all single trials in each class, X^T is the transpose of matrix X and $trace(X)$ is equal to the sum of the diagonal elements of matrix X. In order to factories the composite spatial covariance we have

$$R = R_1 + R_0 = VDV^T \tag{3}$$

where R is the element wise sum of R_1 and R_0, D is the diagonal matrix of eigenvalues and V is the matrix of eigenvectors. In order to generate the whitening transformation matrix P, we have

$$P = \frac{V^T}{\sqrt{D}} = D^{\frac{-1}{2}} V^T. \tag{4}$$

P transforms the covariance matrices of the two classes as

$$S_1 = PR_1 P^T \tag{5}$$

and

$$S_0 = PR_0 P^T \tag{6}$$

where S_1 and S_0 have the same eigenvectors in U_1 and U_0 and the sum of their respective eigenvalues in Σ_1 and Σ_0 would always be equal to I. So we would have:

$$S_1 = U_1 \Sigma_1 U_1^T \tag{7}$$

and

$$S_0 = U_0 \Sigma_0 U_0^T \tag{8}$$

where $U = U_1 = U_0$ and $\Sigma_1 + \Sigma_0 = I$. The eigenvectors that are corresponding to the greatest eigenvalues for S_1 would correspond to the lowest eigenvalues for S_0 and vice versa. The optimal approach to split variance in the two signal

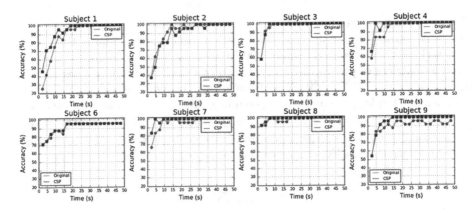

Fig. 4. Comparison of CSP and the original work accuracy results

matrices would be to transform the whitened EEG into the eigenvectors that correspond to the greatest eigenvalues in Σ_1 and Σ_0. The full projection matrix Θ is obtained as

$$\Theta = P^T U \tag{9}$$

where $\Theta \in \mathbb{R}^{N \times N}$, so $\Theta = (\theta_1 \theta_2 \dots \theta_{N-1} \theta_N)$ where $\theta \in \mathbb{R}^N$. Here the first column, θ_1, provides the maximum and minimum variances for class one and two respectively, on the other side, the last column, θ_N, does the opposite. Hence, in order to extract top $m \leq N$ most important spatial filters, $\frac{m}{2}$ columns from each side need to be selected. The projection matrix W is calculated as shown below:

$$W^{-1} = (\theta_1 \dots \theta_{\frac{m}{2}} \theta_{N-\frac{m}{2}+1} \dots \theta_N) \tag{10}$$

Using the projection matrix W, the original raw EEG could be transformed into its uncorrelated components Z by

$$Z = WX. \tag{11}$$

Finally, the original raw EEG, X, could then be reconstructed by $X = W^{-1}Z$.

3.3.2   Independent Component Analysis

The algorithm that was used for the purpose of this work is named FastICA. It is an efficient version of ICA which was firstly introduce in [13]. FastICA algorithm is explained below using the example of EEG data.

Let's assume X denotes the matrix of preprocessed EEG where $X \in \mathbb{R}^{N \times T \times M}$, N is the number of channels (electrodes), T is the number of samples per channel per single trial (sampling rate × single trial time) and M is the number of single trials in the data. Hence $X_i \in \mathbb{R}^{N \times T}$ denotes a two dimensional matrix of ith single trial in X where $1 \leq i \leq M$.

In order to apply ICA to this data, first we need to change its representation a little bit. Consider each $x_{j,z} \in X^i$ for $1 \leq j \leq N$ and $1 \leq z \leq T$ as one

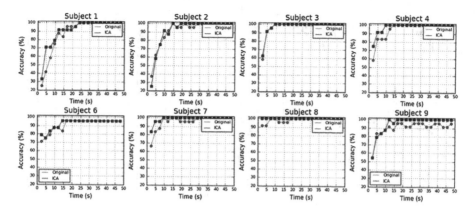

Fig. 5. Comparison of ICA and the original work accuracy results

feature of the data in X_i. This gives us $n = N \times T$ features that each represent one electrode recording at a given time in that single trial. It helps us to change the representation of our preprocessed EEG matrix into a new two dimensional matrix of $X \in \mathbb{R}^{n \times M}$, $x_{i,j} \in X$, $1 \leq i \leq n$ and $1 \leq j \leq M$. Here n rows and M columns corresponding to the number of features (electrode-time) and single trials (samples) respectively. Next, the input data in each row of matrix X must be centered to make its mean equal to zero. It can be done as

$$x_{i,j} \Leftarrow x_{i,j} - \frac{\Sigma_{z=1}^{M} x_{i,z}}{M}. \tag{12}$$

Next, before applying the FastICA algorithm, the data needs to be whitened in order to maximize its non-Gaussian characteristics. This is done by

$$X \Leftarrow VD^{\frac{-1}{2}}V^T X \tag{13}$$

where $VDV^T = E\{XX^T\}$, that means V and D contain the eigenvectors and eigenvalues for the expectation on XX^T. In order to obtain $m \leq n$ independent components, we need to calculate $W \in \mathbb{R}^{m \times n}$, the un-mixing matrix where each row projects X onto an independent component. It can be done by following the pseudocode that follows.

for p in $1 : m$ **do**
    Initialize w_p, a random vector of length n where $||w_p|| = 1$
    while w_p not converged **do**
        $g(y) = tanh(y)$ or $g(y) = ye^{-y^2/2}$
        $w_p \leftarrow \frac{1}{M} Xg(w_p^T X)^T - \frac{1}{M} g'(w_p^T X)w_p$
        $w_p \leftarrow w_p - \Sigma_{j=1}^{p-1} w_p^T w_j w_j$
        $w_p \leftarrow w_p/||w_p||$
    end while
end for

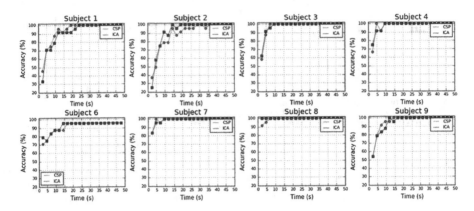

Fig. 6. Comparison of ICA and CSP accuracy results

Next, W can be obtained by

$$W^{-1} = (w_1 \ldots w_m) \tag{14}$$

and finally, independent components matrix, $S \in \mathbb{R}^{m \times M}$, can be calculated by

$$S = WX. \tag{15}$$

4   Results and Discussion

As described earlier, four-fold cross validation was performed in order to estimate the average classification accuracy achieved for each subject. For all Figures in this chapter, the accuracy rate is plotted against the time taken from the user to achieve that. This helps us to compare not only the maximum accuracy achieved in each case but also the time required in order to achieve that. It is also important to mention that the data for subject 5 was excluded from the dataset published by Hoffmann et al.'s work. It leaves us with the eight remaining subjects.

In Fig. 4 the accuracy results of CSP for each subject is plotted in comparison to those of the original work. It is clear that CSP has led to better results for all subjects except subject 2; specially for subject 9, CSP could achieve 100% accuracy rate after only 6 blocks of flashes, while the original work could never exceed 95%. On the other hand, CSP has 16.5% longer data processing time as compared to the original work, which can be an acceptable trade-off for the higher accuracy achieved.

In Fig. 5 the accuracy results of ICA for each subject is plotted in comparison to those of the original work. It is clear that ICA has led to better results for all subjects, even for subject 2. Similar to CSP, ICA could achieve 100% accuracy

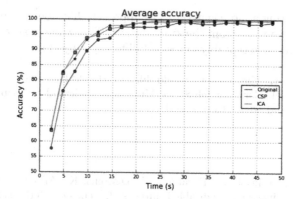

Fig. 7. Comparison of average accuracy results for all three methods across all subjects

rate for subject 9. It is especially interesting to see that using ICA, subject 8's accuracy rate reaches 100% from the first tested block. However, ICA has 43.3% longer data processing time as compared to the original work, this can rise a major concern for the choice of ICA.

In order to have a better comparison between CSP and ICA, Fig. 6 shows their accuracy results in one plot. For most of the subjects, they produce a very similar accuracy rate except that ICA outperforms CSP with regard to subject 2 and 8. Though, ICA's processing time is 23% longer than CSP.

Finally, the average accuracy results for all three methods are plotted together in Fig. 7. It is evident that ICA and CSP have resulted in very similar average accuracies while they have outperformed the original work.

5   Conclusion

In this paper two feature extraction methods, CSP and ICA, were implemented in a P300 based BCI system that was specifically designed for disabled users. The presented data was processed using these two implementations and a comparative analysis took place. It was demonstrated that the implementation of Independent Component Analysis (ICA) and Common Spatial Pattern (CSP) would result in a better feature set than those of raw EEG and hence an improvement in final classification accuracy. Thus, this could be helpful with regards to disabled patients using a faster BCI system that is purposed by this work. It also worth mentioning that despite its better accuracy result, ICA's longer processing time can potentially nullify its advantage over CSP if applied in a real time scenario or processed using an average processor.

There are three possible directions for further improvement of this work. First, to use a more data oriented or learning approach to choose the frequency bandpass that the data is going to be filtered on. Second, to replace winsorizing with a more state of the art outlier detection, and finally, by looking into the possibility of creating a more generalizable approach that does not require training and testing data to be from the same subject. This would lead to generalized classifiers that works acceptably across all different subjects.

Acknowledgement. The authors would like to thank Dr. Jeremiah Deng, Mr. Abdolkarim H. Maleki, Dr. Marzieh Shiva, Mr. Shane Little and Mr. Sebastian Moore for their supports and advice to this work.

References

1. Hoffmann, U., Vesin, J.-M., Ebrahimi, T., Diserens, K.: An efficient P300-based brain computer interface for disabled subjects. J. Neurosci. Methods **167**, 115–125 (2008)
2. Wolpaw, J., Birbaumer, N., McFarland, D., Pfurtscheller, G., Vaughan, T.: Brain-computer interfaces for communication and control. Clin. Neurophysiol. **113**, 767–791 (2002). Official journal of the International Federation of Clinical Neurophysiology
3. Lebedev, M., Nicolelis, M.: Brain-machine interfaces: past, present and future. Trends in Neurosci. **29**, 536–546 (2006)
4. Sutton, S., Braren, M., Zubin, J., John, E.: Evoked-potential correlates of stimulus uncertainty. Science **150**, 1187–1188 (1965). (New York, N.Y.)
5. Farwell, L., Donchin, E.: Talking off the top of your head: toward a mental prosthesis utilizing event-related brain potentials. Electroencephalogr. Clin. Neurophysiol. **70**, 510–523 (1988)
6. Sellers, E.W., Donchin, E.: A P300-based brain-computer interface: initial tests by ALS patients. Clin. Neurophysiol. **117**, 538–548 (2006)
7. Lotte, F., Congedo, M., Lécuyer, A., Lamarche, F., Arnaldi, B.: A review of classification algorithms for EEG-based brain-computer interfaces. J. Neural Eng. **4**, R1 (2007)
8. Grosse-Wentrup, M., Buss, M.: Multiclass common spatial patterns and information theoretic feature extraction. IEEE Trans. Bio Med. Eng. **55**, 1991–2000 (2008)
9. Ramoser, H., Müller-Gerking, J., Pfurtscheller, G.: Optimal spatial filtering of single trial EEG during imagined hand movement. IEEE Trans. Rehabil. Eng. **8**, 441–446 (2001). A publication of the IEEE Engineering in Medicine and Biology Society
10. Jutten, C., Herault, J.: Blind separation of sources, part I: an adaptive algorithm based on neuromimetic architecture. Signal Process. **24**, 1–10 (1991)
11. Comon, P.: Independent component analysis, a new concept? Signal Process. **36**, 287–314 (1994)
12. Wang, Y., Gao, S., Gao, X.: Common spatial pattern method for channel selection in motor imagery based brain-computer interface. In: 27th Annual Conference of IEEE Engineering in Medicine and Biology, pp. 5392–5395 (2005)
13. Hyvarinen, A.: Fast and robust fixed-point algorithms for independent component analysis. IEEE Trans. Neural Netw. **10**, 626–634 (1999)

Thermal Stratification Prediction at Lake Trevallyn

Ashfaqur Rahman[1]([✉]), Philip Smethurst[1], Michael Attard[3], and Rob Dunne[2]

[1] CSIRO, Sandy Bay, Australia
ashfaqur.rahman@csiro.au
[2] CSIRO, Sydney, Australia
[3] NRM North, Launceston, Australia

Abstract. Thermal stratification refers to difference of temperature across water column and can act as a proxy of algal bloom. Algal bloom is a problem in Lake Trevallyn in Launceston, Tasmania. Administrators are interested in finding the causes of algal bloom and in prediction of such events in Lake Trevallyn. The results presented in this paper are the findings from a study to predict thermal stratification in Lake Trevallyn using a machine learning based approach.

Keywords: Algal bloom prediction · Thermal stratification · Lake Trevallyn

1 Introduction

Lake Trevallyn (also known as Trevallyn Dam) is a concrete gravity dam that stores and provides water for hydroelectricity [1]. The lake is located on the lower South Esk River in Launceston, Tasmania (Fig. 1(a)) and is operated by Hydro Tasmania. The water from the lake is mainly directed towards Trevallyn Power Station and the rest mainly pass through Cataract Gorge (in the form of spills mainly). The storage is 6 km long, approximately 200 m wide and has an average depth of around 15 m [1].

Lake Trevallyn is an important source of drinking water for Launceston. It is also extensively used for recreational activities including swimming, water skiing, fishing and kayaking, and is supportive of a commercial eel fishery [1]. In recent years presence of toxic algal bloom became apparent in Lake Trevallyn. The bloom persisted for a while and impacted upon drinking water sourced from Lake Trevallyn by introducing taste and odour compounds. It also posed health concerns for recreational users of the lake and required the relocation of a major recreational event to another location.

In subsequent years, a comprehensive monitoring program was established by NRM North to determine the major drivers of bloom establishment and provide up-to-date information to stakeholders in relation to the bloom status. Following a comprehensive study, the key driver of bloom formation in Lake Trevallyn was hypothesised as being the formation of thermal stratification.

Thermal stratification refers to the change of temperature across the water column and is an indication of stationary water body that is ideal for algal bloom. During summer months, surface water is relatively warm and light. As a result the chance of natural movement across the water body is low compared to winter months. This results in stationary water body in absence of other influence. This creates an ideal environment

© Springer International Publishing AG 2017
U Kang et al. (Eds.): PAKDD 2017 Workshops, LNAI 10526, pp. 51–55, 2017.
DOI: 10.1007/978-3-319-67274-8_5

for algal bloom. During winter months water remains stationary as well. However cold weather is not suitable to algal growth.

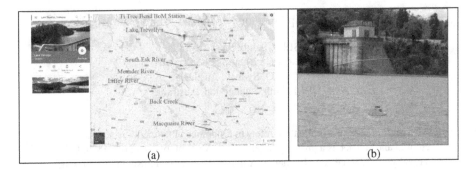

Fig. 1. Lake Trevallyn: (a) Google Map view, (b) Remote Senor Buoy

Early indication of thermal stratification can thus act as a good proxy for algal bloom. The monitoring program thus deployed remote sensor buoys (Fig. 1(b)) near the Lake Trevallyn to continuously monitor water column temperature data that provided an opportunity to assess in more detail the effect of environmental factors on thermal stratification. The buoy was placed near the dam wall and used to monitor in situ water temperature at 1 m intervals starting at the surface extending down to 10 m. The research presented in this paper are some early results on predicting thermal stratification in Lake Trevallyn.

In this preliminary analysis presented in the paper, we aimed at developing a machine learning model that can predict temperature difference across the water column at Lake Trevallyn. A number of weather and natural variables can influence the stationarity of the water body [1–5] and the purpose of the machine learning model is to express temperature difference as a function of these variables.

2 Variables Influencing Stratification

The variables that commonly influence stationarity of water body includes: air temperature, relative humidity, wind direction, wind speed, global radiation, net radiation, air pressure, stream/river flow, and rainfall. Following is a map of Lake Trevallyn (Fig. 1(a)). The nearest BoM station is at Ti Tree Bend. We were able to collect data on air temperature, humidity, wind speed and direction from this BoM station. Data on solar radiation, air pressure, and rainfall were collected from SILO [7]. It can be observed from the map that water from South Esk River flows to Lake Trevallyn. We were unable to collect any flow data on this part of the South Esk River. We thus utilised the flow information from rivers that runs into South Esk River. We collated flow data on Meander River, Liffey River, Back Creek, Macquaire River, and South Esk near Macquaire River.

Data on temperature across the water body was collected from a remote sensor buoy deployed near the Lake Trevallyn dam wall [1]. The buoy used to monitor in situ water temperature at 1 m intervals starting at the surface extending down to 10 m.

3   Results and Analysis

Initially we planned to formulate a machine learning approach to predict the temperature difference directly as a function of the abovementioned influence variables. However, most of the natural and weather variables have little correlations with the temperature difference. Figure 2 shows correlations between the influence variables and water column temperature difference at between 0.5 m (surface) to 10 m depth. Note that the correlation scores are very small and hence implies little relevance to the influence variables directly. This will lead to poor prediction accuracy.

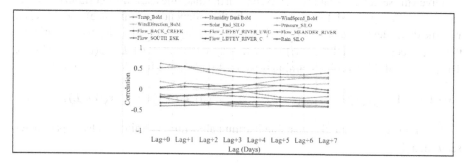

Fig. 2. Correlation between influence variables and water column temperature difference: surface to 10 m depth. Up to 7 days lag is considered.

As an alternative approach we thus tried to develop machine learning models to predict temperature across the water column. The difference between predicted water column temperatures can be computed as proxy for thermal stratification. As first step, we computed the correlations between the influence variables and water column temperature to identify relevant influence variables at Lake Trevallyn. Figure 3 shows the correlation results for up to 7 days lag at water column depth 0.5 m and 10 m. Considering a 0.5 minimum limit for good correlation, the following variables are selected: air temperature, humidity, solar radiation, flow data on Meander River and Liffey River. As the data collected on Macquaire River had significant percentage of missing values, we did not use this variable in further analysis.

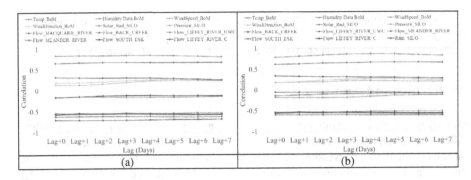

Fig. 3. Correlation between influence variables and water column temperature difference: (a) surface to 0.5 m depth, (b) surface to 10 m depth. Up to 7 days lag is considered.

Given the selected variables we next design the machine learning algorithm to predict temperature a day ahead. Let $x_1, x_2, \ldots, x_N$ be the independent (influence) variables and y be the dependent variable. Considering a lag of L days for each independent variable, the input vector will be like: $x_1(i), \ldots, x_1(i+L), x_2(i), \ldots, x_2(i+L), x_N(i) \ldots, x_N(i+L)$. The purpose of the machine learning model is to develop a function f such that

$$y(i+L+1) \approx f_\theta\big(x_1(i), \ldots, x_1(i+L), x_2(i), \ldots, x_2(i+L), x_N(i) \ldots, x_N(i+L)\big) \tag{1}$$

Given historical data, the machine learning algorithm is trained to learn parameter set $\hat\theta$ such that

$$\overset{min}{\hat\theta} \sum_i y(i+L+1) - f_{\hat\theta}\big(x_1(i), \ldots, x_1(i+L), x_2(i), \ldots, x_2(i+L), x_N(i), \ldots, x_N(i+L)\big) \tag{2}$$

We considered lag days of 4 days and trained a linear and non-linear regression (SVR) algorithm. We predicted the temperature a day ahead. The SVR regression results were poor and we concentrated on linear regression. We trained models on data from

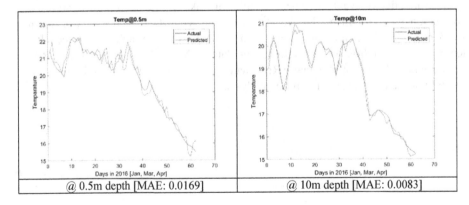

Fig. 4. Day ahead temperature prediction

2014 and 2015. We tested the predictions on 2016 data. Figure 4 presents the day ahead temperature prediction results on test data at 0.5 m and 10 m depth. The temperature difference between depth 0.5 m to 10 m depth from predicted temperature is presented in Fig. 5.

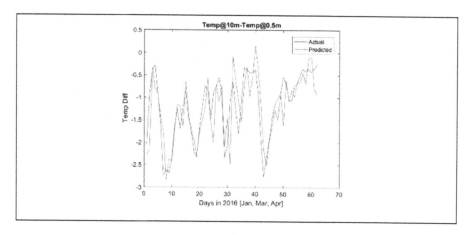

Fig. 5.   Temperature difference between predicted temperatures: 0.5 m and 10 m depth. [MAE: 0.0187]

4   Conclusion

In this paper we present some preliminary finding from our research on predicting thermal stratification in Lake Trevallyn as a proxy of algal bloom. The one day ahead prediction shows promising signs and in future we aim to extend this analysis to multiple days/months ahead prediction.

References

1. NRM North, "Lake Trevallyn Algal Monitoring Program," August 2014. http://www.nrmnorth.org.au/reports. Accessed Dec 2016
2. Lake stratification. https://en.wikipedia.org/wiki/Lake_stratification. Accessed Dec 2016
3. Statistical quantification of the effect of thermal stratification on patterns of dispersion in a freshwater zooplankton community, link: http://link.springer.com/article/10.1007%2Fs10452-005-9021-3#/page-1. Accessed Dec 2016
4. Predicting the onset of thermal stratification in shallow inland waterbodies, link: http://link.springer.com/article/10.1007/s00027-009-8063-3#/page-2. Accessed Dec 2016
5. Mathematical prediction of thermal stratification of lake ostrovo (vegoritis), Greece, link: http://onlinelibrary.wiley.com/doi/10.1029/WR022i011p01590/pdf. Accessed Dec 2016
6. Stratification of lakes, link: http://onlinelibrary.wiley.com/doi/10.1029/2006RG000210/epdf. Accessed Dec 2016
7. SILO climate data, https://www.longpaddock.qld.gov.au/silo/, Accessed Dec 2016

BDM

Development of a Software Vulnerability Prediction Web Service Based on Artificial Neural Networks

Cagatay Catal[✉], Akhan Akbulut, Ecem Ekenoglu, and Meltem Alemdaroglu

Department of Computer Engineering, Istanbul Kültür University,
34156 Bakirköy, Istanbul, Turkey
c.catal@iku.edu.tr
http://www.cagataycatal.com

Abstract. Detecting vulnerable components of a web application is an important activity to allocate verification resources effectively. Most of the studies proposed several vulnerability prediction models based on private and public datasets so far. In this study, we aimed to design and implement a software vulnerability prediction web service which will be hosted on Azure cloud computing platform. We investigated several machine learning techniques which exist in Azure Machine Learning Studio environment and observed that the best overall performance on three datasets is achieved when Multi-Layer Perceptron method is applied. Software metrics values are received from a web form and sent to the vulnerability prediction web service. Later, prediction result is computed and shown on the web form to notify the testing expert. Training models were built on datasets which include vulnerability data from Drupal, Moodle, and PHPMyAdmin projects. Experimental results showed that Artificial Neural Networks is a good alternative to build a vulnerability prediction model and building a web service for vulnerability prediction purpose is a good approach for complex systems.

Keywords: Vulnerability prediction · Artificial neural networks · Machine learning · Web service · Prediction model · Vulnerabilities

1 Introduction

Software security is an important consideration that must be met during the software development life cycle. Although there are many techniques and tools for software security, software security vulnerabilities are still very common. On May 13, 2015, the U.S. Food and Drug Administration (FDA) published an alert about computerized infusion pumps, which can be programmed remotely by malicious Internet users to modify the dosage of therapeutic drugs. The FDA suggested several actions be taken by hospitals using these systems in order to secure them. For example, it recommended that ports 20 (FTP) and 23 (TELNET) be closed to avoid unauthorized access to the infusion pumps. As can be

© Springer International Publishing AG 2017
U Kang et al. (Eds.): PAKDD 2017 Workshops, LNAI 10526, pp. 59–67, 2017.
DOI: 10.1007/978-3-319-67274-8_6

seen from this recent incident, software security vulnerabilities are quite dangerous for software-intensive systems. Cyber-attacks use these unknown vulnerabilities, and sometimes those vulnerabilities are only detected many years later. The Open Web Application Security Project (OWASP) describes the top 10 threats for web applications — namely, injection, broken authentication and session management, cross-site scripting (XSS), insecure direct object references, security misconfiguration, sensitive data exposure, missing function level access control, cross-site request forgery, using components with known vulnerabilities, and unvalidated redirects and forwards. In this study, our aim is to create a web service for software vulnerability prediction that is based on machine learning algorithms and that will be published on the Azure cloud platform. Azure Machine Learning Studio's environment was used during experiments, and several machine learning models based on Area Under ROC Curve (AUC) evaluation parameter was investigated. After selecting the best model, this model was deployed as a web service, and a web form was implemented to obtain software metrics. The following metrics were used as features of the models: Cyclomatic complexity, lines of code, lines of code (non-HTML), number of functions, maximum nesting complexity, Halstead's volume, total external calls, fan-in, fan-out, internal functions called, external functions called, external calls to functions. In addition to these independent variables, a dependent variable called IsVulnerable was used. This variable indicates whether the module had a vulnerability report or not. Therefore, the problem is considered as a two-class classification problem. Three datasets from three different projects were used during the experiments. These datasets include 223 vulnerabilities in total. These vulnerabilities were divided into five categories namely, code injection, cross-site request forgery (CSRF), cross-site scripting (XSS), path disclosure, and authorization issues & other types. While PHPMyAdmin dataset has 75 vulnerabilities, Moodle has 51 and Drupal dataset has 97 vulnerabilities. The following machine learning algorithms in Azure ML Studio were investigated: The averaged perceptron method, the Bayes point machine, boosted decision tree, decision forest, decision jungle, locally deep support vector machine, logistic regression, support vector machine, neural network model. We calculated the average AUC values of these algorithms for three datasets and reported that neural network provides the best performance. The next section shows the related work, Sect. 3 explains methodology, Sect. 4 details the results, and Sect. 5 provides the conclusion and future work.

2   Related Work

Taint analysis was used in conjunction with data mining [1]. Candidate vulnerabilities are detected with taint analysis and false positives are identified by using data mining technique. An approach was developed to make static analysis tools learn to detect vulnerabilities by applying machine learning [2]. It was shown that SVM-based prediction model using code metrics is capable of detection of vulnerabilities for Android applications [3]. A model based on N-gram analysis and feature selection technique was developed to predict vulnerable components [4]. Static and dynamic code attributes were applied to detect vulnerabilities in web applications [5]. They reported that semi-supervised learning is preferable when vulnerability data is limited. A new prediction model was implemented by using CERT-C Secure Coding Standard [6]. An approach was suggested using metrics in conjunction with text mining [7]. Their model builds six classifiers and then, a meta classifier processes the output of these six classifiers. Text mining based models were reported to be better than metrics-based models without considering the component sizes [8]. It was concluded that software metrics-based models are comparable to models using text mining. A Proactive Cybersecurity System (PCS) which collects big data from several data sources, processes this data, and identifies potential attacks before they occur was introduced [9]. It was shown that machine learning approach is effective to detect vulnerabilities [10]. It was explained that the number of misclassified bugs is very high and classification of bugs as vulnerabilities is not effective [11]. A vulnerability dataset which has 223 vulnerabilities was prepared [12]. Researchers applied Random Forests algorithm and reported that models using text mining is better than models using metrics in terms of recall parameter. A model was presented based on machine learning to predict the vulnerabilities [13]. Terms in the source code are taken into account and their associated frequencies are noted. It was reported that complexity metrics have correlation with security vulnerabilities [14,15]. Researchers applied logistic regression technique and analyzed the relationship of developer activity, complexity, and code churn with software security vulnerabilities [15]. Decision trees were used to predict the vulnerabilities by using complexity, cohesion, and coupling metrics [16]. It was reported that traditional metrics such as complexity have a weak correlation between vulnerabilities for Windows Vista [17]. Researchers also analyzed the SQL hotspots which are locations having many SQL statements and showed that a file having more SQL hotspots has higher probability to have vulnerability [18]. The correlation between include statements and vulnerabilities was analyzed [19]. A technique based on dependency graph was developed for vulnerability prediction [20]. Researchers built models based on features related to the sanitization and data flow [21,22]. The correlation between vulnerability density and code metrics was analyzed on PHP applications [23]. Static analysis alerts were used to build vulnerability prediction models [24]. It was investigated whether fault prediction models can be used for vulnerability prediction or not [25]. It was concluded that fault prediction models provide similar results as vulnerability prediction models. Researchers studied vulnerability prediction models on Windows operating system and reported that the model using source code level metrics is not accurate [26].

3   Methodology

Azure Machine Learning Studio was used during all experiments. Figure 1 shows a graphical representation of the experiment we created for the Drupal dataset is depicted.

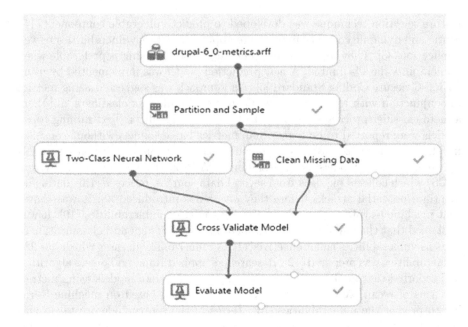

Fig. 1. Experimental design on Azure ML studio

We changed the dataset component for the other experiments. In this figure, we see only two-class neural network algorithms, but we also investigated the performance of the other available machine learning algorithms. The other algorithms we analyzed are shown in Fig. 2.

During our experiments, we applied a 3-fold cross-validation evaluation approach and then, we calculated the AUC parameter's value to judge the performance of each algorithm. Although acceptable AUC values might change based on the investigated problem and domain, the general guideline can be shown as follows:

- 0.90-1.00 Excellent
- 0.80-0.90 Good
- 0.70-0.80 Fair
- 0.60-0.70 Poor
- 0.50-0.60 Fail

However, most of the time, we are unable to reach to the values like 0.90 and 0.80. Therefore, generally values over 0.70 are acceptable for most of the problems in software engineering discipline. In Fig. 3, we show our multi-layer perceptron-based vulnerability prediction model. Our input layer has 13 neurons, hidden layer has three neurons, and output layer has only one neuron. We investigated the impact of the number of neurons in the hidden layer, but the best value was calculated when three was preferred. Output layer indicates whether the module

⊿ Initialize Model

　　⊿ Classification

Multiclass Decision Forest
Multiclass Decision Jungle
Multiclass Logistic Regression
Multiclass Neural Network
One-vs-All Multiclass
Two-Class Averaged Perceptron
Two-Class Bayes Point Machine
Two-Class Boosted Decision Tree
Two-Class Decision Forest
Two-Class Decision Jungle
Two-Class Locally-Deep Support Vector Machine
Two-Class Logistic Regression
Two-Class Neural Network
Two-Class Support Vector Machine

Fig. 2. Algorithms in Azure ML studio

will be vulnerable or not. Input layer includes several software metrics calculated from the source code of the web application.

The following methods were analyzed in the experiments:

– Averaged perceptron: This is a very basic form of a neural network and very useful for linearly detachable patterns.
– Bayes point machine: This method is a Bayesian approximation approach.
– Boosted decision tree: Ensemble of trees is created for the prediction.
– Decision forest: Random decision forest algorithm is applied.
– Decision jungle: This is a recent extension to decision forests. It includes an ensemble of decision directed acyclic graphs.
– Locally deep support vector machine: This is a non-linear support vector machine classifier.
– Logistic regression: This is a well-known statistical method used for supervised classification.
– Support vector machine: This is support vector machine algorithm.
– Neural network module: This is multi-layer perceptron implementation.

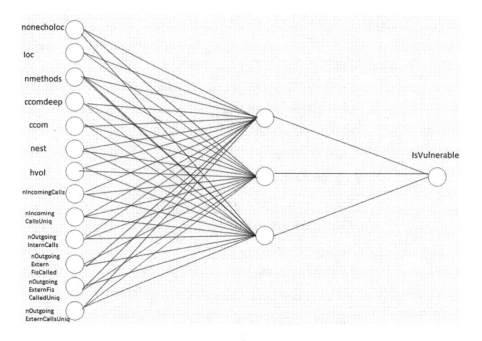

Fig. 3. Our neural network based prediction model

4   Experimental Results

We applied several algorithms on Drupal, Moodle, and PHPMyAdmin datasets. We applied 3-fold cross-validation validation approach. Result of the algorithms are shown in Table 1. For all the datasets, Neural Network achieved a performance larger than 0.70 and this indicates that neural network is a good approach for vulnerability prediction studies. In addition to this algorithm, Bayes point machine, and Logistic Regression provides good performance. We calculated the average results of these algorithms on three datasets. According to these average calculations, the best performance is achieved with Neural Network algorithm. Figure 4 depicts these results. After this observation, we implemented our prediction web service based on this algorithm. Web service was easily built in Azure Machine Learning Studio environment and deployed in Azure cloud. After building the web service on the cloud platform, we designed a user interface form to receive the inputs for the proposed model. These inputs are metrics calculated with a software metrics calculation tool. Once these inputs are sent to the web service, the prediction result is computed in the web service and the result is again returned to the web form to inform the user. While Random Forest algorithm was reported a good algorithm in previous studies [19], its performance was not good according to Table 1. This might be related to the implementation of the algorithm on two platforms (Azure ML Studio and Weka) and the configuration parameters. We did not optimize the parameters and decided to

Table 1. Performance results

Algorithms	Drupal	Moodle	PHPMyAdmin
Avg. Perceptron	0.794	0.632	0.702
Bayes Machine	0.768	0.730	0.742
Decision Tree	0.801	0.644	0.609
Decision Forest	0.786	0.488	0.573
Decision Jungle	0.799	0.631	0.630
Deep SVM	0.800	0.666	0.680
Logistic Regression	0.795	0.755	0.655
Neural Network	0.766	0.811	0.718
SVM	0.800	0.594	0.605

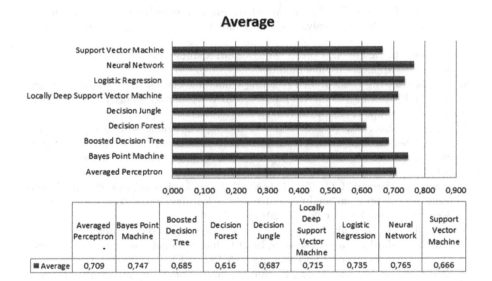

	Averaged Perceptron .	Bayes Point Machine	Boosted Decision Tree	Decision Forest	Decision Jungle	Locally Deep Support Vector Machine	Logistic Regression	Neural Network	Support Vector Machine
■ Average	0,709	0,747	0,685	0,616	0,687	0,715	0,735	0,765	0,666

Fig. 4. Average results of algorithms on three datasets

use them as-is. In the deployed system, we used the published dataset in the literature [19] and we will integrate the system with a metrics calculation tool. After the source code is analyzed by this tool, the prediction web service will predict the vulnerabilities in the software project which is analyzed.

5   Conclusion and Future Work

We investigated several machine learning algorithms for software vulnerability prediction problem and implemented a web service to predict the vulnerabilities. Azure Machine Learning Studio was used during all experiments and the web service was built on the Azure cloud platform. We investigated several classification algorithms for this problem on three datasets: Drupal, Moodle, and PHPMyAdmin. These classification algorithms are averaged perceptron model, Bayes point machine, boosted decision tree, decision forest, decision jungle, locally deep support vector machine, logistic regression, support vector machine, and neural network in Azure ML Studio. According to the performance results on datasets, the best performance is achieved when a multi-layer perceptron model is used. As part of future work, we want to investigate different artificial neural network models (i.e., RBF network, Hopfield network, and Boltzmann machine) in to improve the performance of the proposed model.

References

1. Medeiros, I., Neves, N., Correia, M.: Detecting and removing web application vulnerabilities with static analysis and data mining. IEEE Trans. Reliab. **65**(1), 54–69 (2016)
2. Medeiros, I., Neves, N., Correia, M.: Dekant: a static analysis tool that learns to detect web application vulnerabilities
3. Scandariato, R., Walden, J.: Predicting vulnerable classes in an android application. In: Proceedings of the 4th International Workshop on Security Measurements and Metrics, pp. 11–16, ACM (2012)
4. Pang, Y., Xue, X., Namin, A.S.: Predicting vulnerable software components through n-gram analysis and statistical feature selection. In: 2015 IEEE 14th International Conference on Machine Learning and Applications (ICMLA), pp. 543–548, IEEE (2015)
5. Shar, L.K., Briand, L.C., Tan, H.B.K.: Web application vulnerability prediction using hybrid program analysis and machine learning. IEEE Trans. Dependable Secure Comput. **12**(6), 688–707 (2015)
6. Yang, J., Ryu, D., Baik, J.: Improving vulnerability prediction accuracy with secure coding standard violation measures. In: 2016 International Conference on Big Data and Smart Computing (BigComp), pp. 115–122, IEEE (2016)
7. Zhang, Y., Lo, D., Xia, X., Xu, B., Sun, J., Li, S.: Combining software metrics and text features for vulnerable file prediction. In: 2015 20th International Conference on Engineering of Complex Computer Systems (ICECCS), pp. 40–49, IEEE (2015)
8. Tang, Y., Zhao, F., Yang, Y., Lu, H., Zhou, Y., Xu, B.: Predicting vulnerable components via text mining or software metrics? an effort-aware perspective. In: 2015 IEEE International Conference on Software Quality, Reliability and Security (QRS), pp. 27–36, IEEE (2015)
9. Chen, H.M., Kazman, R., Monarch, I., Wang, P.: Predicting and fixing vulnerabilities before they occur: a big data approach. In: Proceedings of the 2nd International Workshop on BIG Data Software Engineering, pp. 72–75, ACM (2016)
10. Mokhov, S.A., Paquet, J., Debbabi, M.: Marfcat: fast code analysis for defects and vulnerabilities. In: 2015 IEEE 1st International Workshop on Software Analytics (SWAN), pp. 35–38, IEEE (2015)
11. Wright, J.L., Larsen, J.W., McQueen, M.: Estimating software vulnerabilities: a case study based on the misclassification of bugs in mysql server. In: 2013 Eighth International Conference on Availability, Reliability and Security (ARES), pp. 72–81, IEEE (2013)

12. Walden, J., Stuckman, J., Scandariato, R.: Predicting vulnerable components: software metrics vs text mining. In: IEEE 25th International Symposium on Software Reliability Engineering, pp. 23–33, IEEE (2014)
13. Scandariato, R., Walden, J., Hovsepyan, A., Joosen, W.: Predicting vulnerable software components via text mining. IEEE Trans. Softw. Eng. **40**(10), 993–1006 (2014)
14. Shin, Y., Williams, L.: An empirical model to predict security vulnerabilities using code complexity metrics. In: Proceedings of the Second ACM-IEEE Int'l Symposium on Empirical Software Engineering and Measurement, pp. 315–317, ACM (2008)
15. Shin, Y., Meneely, A., Williams, L., Osborne, J.A.: Evaluating complexity, code churn, and developer activity metrics as indicators of software vulnerabilities. IEEE Trans. Softw. Eng. **37**(6), 772–787 (2011)
16. Chowdhury, I., Zulkernine, M.: Using complexity, coupling, and cohesion metrics as early indicators of vulnerabilities. J. Syst. Architect. **57**(3), 294–313 (2011)
17. Zimmermann, T., Nagappan, N., Williams, L.: Searching for a needle in a haystack: predicting security vulnerabilities for windows vista. In: 2010 Third International Conference on Software Testing, Verification and Validation, pp. 421–428, IEEE (2010)
18. Smith, B., Williams, L.: Using sql hotspots in a prioritization heuristic for detecting all types of web application vulnerabilities. In: 2011 Fourth IEEE International Conference on Software Testing, Verification and Validation, pp. 220–229, IEEE (2011)
19. Neuhaus, S., Zimmermann, T., Holler, C., Zeller, A.: Predicting vulnerable software components. In: Proceedings of the 14th ACM Conference on Computer and Communications security, pp. 529–540, ACM (2007)
20. Nguyen, V.H., Tran, L.M.S.: Predicting vulnerable software components with dependency graphs. In: Proceedings of the 6th International Workshop on Security Measurements and Metrics, p. 3, ACM (2010)
21. Shar, L.K., Tan, H.B.K., Briand, L.C.: Mining sql injection and cross site scripting vulnerabilities using hybrid program analysis. In: Proceedings of the 2013 International Conference on Software Engineering, pp. 642–651, IEEE Press (2013)
22. Shar, L.K., Tan, H.B.K.: Predicting common web application vulnerabilities from input validation and sanitization code patterns. In: 2012 Proceedings of the 27th IEEE/ACM International Conference on Automated Software Engineering (ASE), pp. 310–313, IEEE (2012)
23. Walden, J., Doyle, M., Welch, G.A., Whelan, M.: Security of open source web applications. In: Proceedings of the 2009 3rd International Symposium on Empirical Software Engineering and Measurement, IEEE Computer Society, pp. 545–553(2009)
24. Gegick, M., Williams, L., Osborne, J., Vouk, M.: Prioritizing software security fortification throughcode-level metrics. In: Proceedings of the 4th ACM Workshop on Quality of Protection, pp. 31–38, ACM (2008)
25. Shin, Y., Williams, L.: Can traditional fault prediction models be used for vulnerability prediction? Empirical Softw. Eng. **18**(1), 25–59 (2013)
26. Morrison, P., Herzig, K., Murphy, B., Williams, L.: Challenges with applying vulnerability prediction models. In: Proceedings of the 2015 Symposium and Bootcamp on the Science of Security, p. 4, ACM (2015)

Diversification Heuristics in Bees Swarm Optimization for Association Rules Mining

Youcef Djenouri[1]([✉]), Zineb Habbas[2], Djamel Djenouri[3], and Marco Comuzzi[1]

[1] Ulsan National Institute of Science and Technology, Ulsan, Republic of Korea
{ydjenouri,mcomuzzi}@unist.ac.kr
[2] University of Lorraine, Metz, France
zineb.habbas@univ-lorraine.fr
[3] DTISI, CERIST, Algiers, Algeria
ddjenouri@acm.org

Abstract. Association rules mining is becoming more challenging with the large transactional databases typical of modern times. Conventional exact algorithms for association rules mining struggle to cope with very large databases, especially in terms of run-time performance. To address this problem, several evolutionary and swarm intelligence-based approaches have been proposed. One of these is *HBSO-TS*, which is a hybrid approach combining Bees Swarm Optimization with Tabu Search and has been shown to outperform other state-of-the art bio-inspired approaches. The main drawback of *HBSO-TS* is that while the intensification is improved using Tabu Search, the diversification remains unchanged compared to *BSO-ARM*, i.e., the first approach proposed in the literature using Bees Swarm Optimization for association rules mining. To ensure a better balance between intensification and diversification, this paper proposes two new heuristics for determining the search area of the bees. We conducted experimental evaluation on well known data instances to show that both heuristics improve the performance of *HBSO-TS*. Moreover, we show the usefulness of our heuristics in the special case of mining association rules from diversified data, as in the case of Weblog mining.

Keywords: Association rules mining · Swarm intelligence · Diversification strategy · Weblog mining

1 Introduction

Association Rules Mining (ARM) is a well studied techniques in data mining. It aims to extract frequent patterns, associations or causal structures among sets of items from a given transactional database. Formally, the ARM problem is stated as follows: let T be a set of m transactions $\{t_1, t_2, \ldots, t_m\}$ representing a transactional database, and I be a set of n different items or attributes $\{i_1, i_2, \ldots, i_n\}$. An association rule is an implication of the form $X \rightarrow Y$ where $X \subset I$, $Y \subset I$, and $X \cap Y = \emptyset$. The itemset X is called antecedent, while the itemset Y is called consequent and the rule means that X implies Y.

© Springer International Publishing AG 2017
U Kang et al. (Eds.): PAKDD 2017 Workshops, LNAI 10526, pp. 68–78, 2017.
DOI: 10.1007/978-3-319-67274-8_7

Two basic parameters are commonly used for measuring usefulness of association rules, namely the *support* and the *confidence* of a rule. The support of an itemset $I' \subseteq I$ is the number of transactions containing I' in a database. The support of a rule $X \rightarrow Y$ is the support of $X \cup Y$ and the confidence of a rule is $\frac{support(X \cup Y)}{support(X)}$. ARM aims at extracting from a given database all interesting rules, that is, rules with support $\geq MinSup$ and confidence $\geq MinConf$, where $MinSup$ and $MinConf$ are two thresholds predefined by users.

Many exact algorithms have been designed for solving the ARM problem, e.g., Apriori [5], FPGrowth [4] and Eclat [6]. When these methods are applied to extremely large data, such as the ones existing on the Web, the ARM process becomes extremely time consuming. Hence, several bio-inspired methods have been proposed to mainly reduce the run-time. Some algorithms are based on evolutionary algorithms, such as genetic algorithms [8,9], while others are grounded on swarm intelligence, such as PSOARM [10], which uses particle swarm optimization.

In this paper we focus on the application of Bees Swarm Optimization, i.e., a particular bio-inspired technique, to the ARM problem. Bees Swarm Optimization for ARM has been introduced in [1], where an approach called *BSO-ARM* is proposed. More recently, a hybrid approach called *HBSO-TS* has been proposed in [2], which combines BSO with Tabu Search. In *HBSO-TS*, the bees are distributed among different search spaces by using a given determination strategy, according to the *BSO-ARM* algorithm. However, the bees explore their regions by using the tabu search strategy. The experiments reported in [2] confirm that *HBSO-TS* outperforms other state-of-the-art ARM algorithms in terms of the resulting rules quality.

The main drawback of *BSO-ARM*, however, is that the tabu search strategy tends to increase considerably the intensification step, compared to the diversification step. To ensure a better balance between intensification and diversification, this paper proposes two new extended versions of *HBSO-TS*, called *HBSO-TS+D1* and *HBSO-TS+D2*, which consider two different diversification heuristics DT1 and DT2, respectively. These new algorithms have been implemented and tested on standard benchmarks to determine experimentally which is the best one. The results show that the first heuristic *HBSO-TS+D1* is better than the second one and in all cases the two heuristics improve the results yielded by *HBSO-TS*.

HBSO-TS+D1, that is, the best heuristic determined experimentally, is then evaluated on Weblog data instances. The Weblog application is considered as an example of extracting association rules from very large databases. The results of our evaluation show that *HBSO-TS+D1* outperform other ARM approaches that have been applied in the past to Weblogs.

The remainder of the paper is organized as follows: Sect. 2 discusses related work. Section 3 recalls the principle of *BSO-ARM*. Section 4 presents the two new search area heuristics *D1* and *D2* which lead to the design of *HBSO-TS+D1* and *HBSO-TS+D2*. The performance evaluation is described in Sect. 5, and finally, Sect. 6 concludes the paper.

2   Related Work

In the literature, many exact algorithms for generating association rules have been proposed. Exact approaches become inefficient with large databases, such as the one resulting from fast development of the Web. In order to deal with large data sets in a reasonable time, bio-inspired meta-heuristics have been widely applied to the ARM problem. Particularly, the application of genetic algorithms (GAs) to ARM problem is extensively studied in the literature. The first genetic algorithm for ARM (GAR) is proposed in [9]. The main limit of this algorithm is the inefficient representation of the individuals. Many genetic algorithms using an improved representation of the solutions have been proposed, such as ARMGA [7] and AGA [8]. The two major differences between the ARMGA and AGA are the mutation and crossover operators. In [3], the authors propose a comparative study between genetic and memetic algorithms for association rules mining. The experimental study reveals that the memetic algorithm outperforms the genetic algorithm in terms of quality of the rules discovered.

Particle swarm optimization (PSO) is another meta-heuristic largely applied to ARM. In [10], a new ARM algorithm based on PSO is proposed. The neighborhood space is found by moving front and back points of each particle. Although this algorithm outperforms AGA, the search based on front and back points gives a large number of neighborhoods, which favors the intensification of the search as compared to the diversification. To overcome this, in [1,2], two algorithms based on BSO have been proposed that avoid the risk of generating false rules and that solve the admissibility problem by improving the representation of the solution and the fitness function. These algorithms, however, suffer from the diversification issue due to the determination of search area strategy used. In this present paper, an improvement of these two algorithms is proposed in the form of two new intelligent heuristics to determine the search area strategies.

3   BSO-ARM Algorithm

Bees Swarm Optimization for solving ARM problem (BSO-ARM) has been first proposed in [1]. Here, we present the main principle of this algorithm by referring to Algorithm 1.

The initial bee *BeeInit* creates the reference solution named *Sref* and saves it in a Tabu list (Lines 1–2). From *Sref*, a set of k regions $R = \{S_{R1}, S_{R2}, \ldots, S_{Rk}\}$ is determined thanks to a procedure for the determination of regions (Line 4). After that, each bee b_i is assigned to S_{Ri} to explore this region using *LocalSearch* (Lines 5–8). Finally, the communication between bees is performed via *Table Dance*, to elect the best solution that becomes the reference solution for the next iteration (Line 9).

The main principles of BSO-ARM can be synthesized as follows:

- **Evaluation of the solution:** A solution s of BSO-ARM is a vector of n elements, where the ith element is set to 1 if the ith item belongs to the

---

Algorithm 1. BSO-ARM algorithm

Input: A transactional data base T
Begin
1: $Sref \leftarrow$ **Initial_Solution**;
2: **while** non stop **do**
3:    $TabuList \leftarrow Sref$
4:    **FindSearchRegion** $(Sref, k, S_{R1}, S_{R2}, \ldots, S_{Rk})$
5:    **for** each bee i **do**
6:        **LocalSearch** $(S_{Ri}, BestSol_i)$
7:        TableDance $\leftarrow BestSol_i$
8:    **end for**
9:    $Sref \leftarrow$ **BestSolution(Table Dance)**;
10: **end while**
11: **End**

---

antecedent part of a given rule. It is set to 2 if the item appears in the consequent part of the rule. Finally, it is set to 0 if such item does not appear in the rule. The evaluation of s is the sum of both the support and the confidence of the rule associated to it.

- **Determination of regions:** The aim of the procedure **FindSearchRegion** in Algorithm 1 is to divide the space of solutions into k disjoint regions where k is the number of bees. Given the reference solution $Sref$, in order to ensure the diversification characteristic of BSO, the parameter $Flip$ is used. Indeed, k disjoint solutions are generated where the ith solution is obtained by changing successfully from $Sref$ the bits $\{(1 \times Flip) + i, (2 \times Flip) + i, (3 \times Flip) + i, \ldots n - i\}$.

- **Local Search Process:** The aim of the local search is to explore one region by identifying at each step the neighbors of the given solution. Given the solution s, this operation ensures the intensification by changing only one bit of s at a time.

4   Improved Heuristics for Search Space Exploration

In [2], we have proposed a new algorithm for association rules mining called HBSO-TS. It is an adapted version of BSO-ARM described in the previous section. In HBSO-TS, the exploration of the region of each bee is performed efficiently by using a robust tabu search method, while the determination of the search space is done using the basic strategy described above. Clearly, HBSO-TS improves considerably the intensification step, however, the diversification step remains the same. In order to ensure a better balancing between both intensification and diversification, two new strategies, namely $D1$ and $D2$, are proposed for the determination of search area process.

4.1   HBSO-TS+D1

Principle. In this strategy, each bee k builds its own search area by changing all bits of the solution $Sref$ except one bit. The ith bee keeps the ith bit of $Sref$ and modifies the remaining bit in a random way. This strategy can be used if and only if the number of bees is less than or equal to n, where n is the size of a solution. If the distance between two solutions is the number of different bits, then the distance between the bees and the solution reference is equal to $n-1$.

Algorithm 2 describes more formally this strategy.

Algorithm 2. *First* strategy algorithm

1: **Input** Sref, K (Bees Number)
2: **Ouput**: Bees_Space:Array [1...K][1...n]
3: $i \leftarrow 1$
4: **while** $i < K$ **do**
5:     Sref[i]=Bees_Space[i][i]
6:     **for** $j = 1; j \leq n$; j=j+1 **do**
7:         Sref[j]=change_bit(Bees_Space[i][j])
8:     **end for**
9:     $i \leftarrow i + 1$
10: **end while**
11: **return** Bees_Space

Complexity

Proposition 1. *The complexity of HBSO-TS+D1 is $O(Max\_iter \times K \times n + n \times IMAX\_TS)$, where K is the number of bees, Max_iter is the maximal number of iterations, n is the number of items and $IMAX\_TS$ the maximum number of iterations of tabu search method.*

Proof. First, from $Sref$, the search region of each bee is determined using $D1$ strategy. Thus, K iterations are performed, one for each bee. So, the cost of the copy is $O(n)$, where n is the number of all items in the transactional database. After that, each bee modifies its solution $(n-1)$ times. Therefore, the complexity of the modification is $O(n-1)$. The complete cost of $D1$ strategy is $O(K \times n)$. Then, each bee explores $n \times IMAX\_TS$ neighborhoods where $IMAX\_TS$ is the maximum number of iterations used on tabu search algorithm. In the worst case, this process can be repeated until Max_Iter iterations. Consequently, the complexity is $O(Max\_iter \times K \times n + n \times IMAX\_TS)$.

4.2   HBSO-TS+D2

Principle. Unlike the strategy $D1$, the strategy $D2$ uses a syntactical, instead of random, form to generate the solutions. For this purpose, we associate the notion of weight to each solution. Formally, the weight of a solution $S = a_0 a_1 a_2 \ldots a_{n-1}$ noted $W(S)$, is defined as

$$W(s) = \sum_{i=0}^{n-1} a_i,$$

where n is the size of the solution.

For instance, if we consider the solution $S = 0112211$ then $W(S) = 0 + 1 + 1 + 2 + 2 + 1 + 1 = 6$.

Thanks to this idea, each bit i can generate a solution that has a gap of a given distance with $Sref$. First, the algorithm computes $W(Sref)$. Then, each bee k changes the successive bits of $Sref$ starting from the bit k. Each bee k stops this process when it obtains a solution s which satisfies the constraint:

$$W(s) = W(Sref) - Distance \text{ or } W(s) = W(Sref) + Distance$$

Algorithm 3 describes more formally this strategy.

Algorithm 3. *Second* strategy algorithm

1: **Input**: Sref, K (Bees Number), Distance
2: **output** : Bees_Space:Array [1...k][1...n]
3: Compute Weight(Sref)
4: $i \leftarrow 0$
5: **while** $i < K$ **do**
6:    copy(Sref, Bees_Space[i])
7:    **for** $j = 1$;$j < n$; $j \leftarrow j + +$ **do**
8:      Change_Bit(Bees_Space[i][j])
9:      **if** W(Bees_Space[i]) == W(Sref) - Distance or W(Bees_Space[i]) == W(Sref)+Distance **then**
10:        Accepted(Bees_Space[i]
11:        exit
12:      **end if**
13:    **end for**
14:    $i \leftarrow i + 1$
15: **end while**
16: **return** Bees_Space.

Complexity

Proposition 2. *The complexity of HBSO-TS+D2 is $O(Maxiter \times K \times n \times Distance + n \times IMAX\_TS)$ where K is the number of bees, $Maxiter$ is the maximal number of iterations, n is the number of items, $IMAX\_TS$ the maximum number of iterations of tabu search method and $Distance$ is the given parameter of D2 strategy.*

Proof. First, from $Sref$, the search region of each bee is determined using $D2$ strategy. Thus, K iterations are performed, one for each bee. This strategy first calculates the weight of Sref, whose cost is $O(n)$. Then, K iterations are performed. At each iteration, $Sref$ is copied on one bee, then each solution is changed $Distance$ times (in the worst case). The complexity of this strategy is $O(K \times n \times Distance)$. Then, each bee explores $n \times IMAX\_TS$ neighborhoods where $IMAX\_TS$ is the maximum number of iterations used in the tabu search algorithm. In the worst case, this process can be repeated until Max_Iter iterations. Consequently, the complexity is $O(Maxiter \times K \times n \times Distance + n \times IMAX\_TS)$.

5   Experimental Results

To validate the proposed approaches, several tests have been carried out. Experiments have been conducted on a 4 GB Intel Core I3 machine running Windows 7 and all algorithms are scripted in C++. First, *HBSO-TS+D1* and *HBSO-TS+D2* are compared in order to determine the best heuristic among them using well-known ARM instances [12]. Then, we compare the best identified heuristic *HBSO-TS* with the classical version of *HBSO-TS* proposed in [2]. Finally, the best heuristic is applied on Weblog data instances using the data instance described in [16].

5.1   Comparing the Two Proposed Heuristics

Table 1 presents the solution quality returned by the two algorithms *HBSO-TS-D1* and *HBSO-TS-D2*. The solution quality is computed using the evaluation procedure defined in Sect. 3. The first heuristic outperforms the second one in all cases. In fact, the first heuristic allows to divide efficiently the search space among the bees. These experiments lead us to choose the first algorithm *HBSO-TS-D1* for the remaining experiments.

Table 1. HBSO-TS-D1 Vs HBSO-TS-D2 in terms of solution quality

Number of transactions	HBSO-TS+D1	HBSO-TS+D2
10	0.50	0.04
100	0.53	0.28
1000	0.51	0.26
10000	0.49	0.25
100000	0.50	0.12

5.2 HBSO-TS-D1 Algorithm Performance

In order to compare the improved HBSO-TS version, i.e., HBSO-TS-D1, with the classical HBSO-TS reported in [2], we used the well-known ARM instances described in [12]. Note that the obtained results are the average of 100 executions. Table 2 summarizes the results that we obtained by executing *HBSO-TS-D1* and the *HBSO-TS* in terms of the fitness function described above. Note that n is the number of items and m is the number of transactions in a database. *HBSO-TS-D1* outperforms the classical *HBSO-TS* using the large data sets. Indeed, the average fitness does not exceed 0.70. These interesting results are reached mainly thanks to the carefully chosen strategy in the determination search area.

Table 2. Fitness quality of the HBSO-TS-D1 compared to the classical HBSO-TS

Dataset Name	(m, n)	HBSO-TS+D1	HBSO-TS
Bolts	(40, 8)	1.0	1.0
Sleep	(56, 8)	1.0	1.0
Pollution	(60, 16)	1.0	1.0
Basket ball	(96, 5)	0.97	0.97
IBM Quest Standard	(1000, 40)	0.94	0.94
Quake	(2178, 4)	1.0	1.0
Chess	(3196, 75)	0.90	0.90
Mushroom	(8124, 119)	0.78	0.75
Pumbs_star	(40385, 7116)	0.83	0.72
BMS-WebView-1	(59602, 497)	0.75	0.55
BMS-WebView-2	(77512, 3340)	0.80	0.70
Korasak	(80769, 7116)	0.79	0.65
retail	(88162, 16469)	0.78	0.62
Connect	(100000, 999)	0.80	0.50
BMP POS	(515597, 1657)	0.82	0.47

5.3 Evaluation with Weblog Data

Weblogs are unstructured and heterogeneous data created to share information, opinions, hobbies on the Web by different users. Extracting relevant knowledge from Weblog is a challenging task. Recently, a considerable number of research works have investigated the issue of extracting relevant association rules from Weblogs, e.g., [14–16]. The main drawback of existing algorithms for association rules mining when applied to Web log mining is the poor quality of the rules returned. Poor rule quality is mainly determined because of diversified data contained in Weblogs.

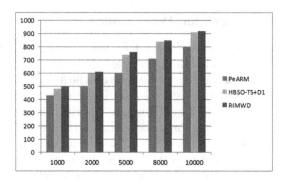

Fig. 1. Runtime (Sec) of the proposed approaches and the state-of-the-art weblog algorithm

Our proposed approach *HBSO-TS-D1* should improve the ability to handle diversified data. Therefore, in order to better validate our diversification heuristic, several experiments have been carried out using Weblog data instances described in [16]. Figure 1 shows the execution time in seconds of *HBSO-TS+D1* compared to the recently proposed approaches RIMWD [16] and PeARM [13], which also focus on applications to Weblog data. We remark that PeARM outperforms HBSO-TS+D1 and RIMWD in terms of runtime no matter the number of Weblog records used, while the runtime of HBSO-TS+D1 and RIMWD are very similar. Figure 2 shows the number of generated satisfied rules of HBSO-TS-D1 compared to RIMWD and Pe-ARM, when the number of Weblog records is set to 10000. According to this figure, we remark that HBSO-TS+D1 outperforms both Pe-ARM and RIMWD in terms of the number of satisfied rules for any minimum support threshold. Moreover, the number of generated satisfied rules is reduced when the minimum support is increased.

By considering these experiments, we can conclude that our approach *HBSO-TS+D1* outperforms the recently developed approach *RIMWD* for Weblog data

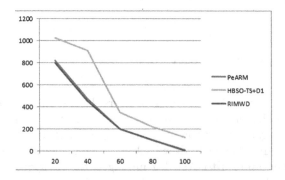

Fig. 2. Number of satisfied rules generated by the proposed approaches and the state-of-the-art weblog algorithm

analysis in terms of both runtime and success rate. Moreover, it outperforms *PeARM* in terms of success rate. These results appear to be very promising and will drive our work in the future to further improve HBSO-TS-D1 to be able to deal with very large and diversified data instances.

6   Conclusions

In this paper, we proposed HBSO-TS+D1 and HBSO-TS+D2, two extended versions of the HBSO-TS algorithm for ARM. The two new versions consider two new heuristics to determine the search area of each bee in order to ensure a better balance between intensification and diversification compared to HBSO-TS. To demonstrate the efficiency of the proposed approach, we carried out several experiments on standard data sets. The experimental process is divided into three main steps. First, the two strategies of determination of the search area are compared in terms of solution quality. The results of this first step revealed that the first strategy (each bee k randomly modifies all the bits of the reference solution except the kth bit) outperforms the second one (using a distance measure between each solution and the reference solution). The second step of the experimental process consists of comparing the improved HBSO-TS algorithm (based on the first strategy to determine the search area) to the classical version of HBSO-TS algorithm. The obtained results show that the improved HBSO-TS outperforms the classical version in terms of rules quality. Finally, to better validate our claim, our approach is applied on diversified data as the case of Weblog mining. The results reveal that *HBSO-TS+D1* outperforms the state of the art weblog mining approaches in terms of success rate and it is very competitive with Pe-ARM compared to runtime. In perspective, we will investigate to parallelize the proposed approaches for dealing with big Weblog data instances.

References

1. Djenouri, Y., Drias, H., Habbas, Z.: Bees swarm optimisation using multiple strategies for association rule mining. Int. J. Bio Inspired Comput. **6**(4), 239–249 (2014)
2. Djenouri, Y., Drias, H., Habbas, Z.: Hybrid intelligent method for association rules mining using multiple strategies. Int. J. Appl. Metaheurist. Comput. (IJAMC) **5**(1), 46–64 (2014)
3. Djenouri, Y., Bendjoudi, A., Nouali-Taboudjemat, N., Habbas, Z.: An improved evolutionary approach for association rules mining. In: Pan, L., Păun, G., Pérez-Jiménez, M.J., Song, T. (eds.) BIC-TA 2014. CCIS, vol. 472, pp. 93–97. Springer, Heidelberg (2014). doi:10.1007/978-3-662-45049-9_16
4. Han, J., Pei, J., Yin, Y.: Mining frequent patterns without candidate generation. ACM Sigmod Rec. **29**(2), 1–12 (2000). ACM
5. Agrawal, R., Srikant, R.: Fast algorithms for mining association rules. In: Proceedings of 20th International Conference on Very Large Data Bases (VLDB), vol. 1215, pp. 487–499, September 1994

6. Zaki, M.J., Parthasarathy, S., Ogihara, M., Li, W.: New algorithms for fast discovery of association rules. In: KDD, vol. 97, pp. 283–286, August 1997
7. Yan, X., Zhang, C., Zhang, S.: Genetic algorithm-based strategy for identifying association rules without specifying actual minimum support. Expert Syst. Appl. **36**(2), 3066–3076 (2009)
8. Wang, M., Zou, Q., Lin, C.: Multi dimensions association rules mining on adaptive genetic algorithm. In: International Conference on Uncertainly Reasoning on Knowledge Engineering. IEEE (2011)
9. Mata, J., Alvarez, J., Riquelme, J.: An evolutionary algorithm to discover numeric association rules. In: Proceedings of the ACM Symposium on Applied Computing (SAC), pp. 590–594 (2002)
10. Kuo, R.J., Chao, C.M., Chiu, Y.T.: Application of particle swarm optimization to association rule mining. J. Appl. Soft Comput. **11**, 326–336 (2011)
11. Zheng, Z., Kohavi, R., Mason, L.: Real world performance of association rule algorithms. Knowl. Disc. Database J. (2001)
12. Goethals, B., Zaki, M.J.: Frequent itemset mining implementations repository (2003). http://fimi.cs.helsinki.fi
13. Gheraibia, Y., Moussaoui, A., Djenouri, Y., Kabir, S., Yin, P.Y., Mazouzi, S.: Penguin search optimisation algorithm for finding optimal spaced seeds. Int. J. Softw. Sci. Comput. Intell. (IJSSCI) **7**(2), 85–99 (2015)
14. Bakariya, B., Thakur, G.S.: An efficient algorithm for extracting high utility itemsets from weblog data. IETE Tech. Rev. **32**(2), 151–160 (2015)
15. Senkul, P., Salin, S.: Improving pattern quality in web usage mining by using semantic information. Knowl. Inf. Syst. **30**(3), 527–541 (2012)
16. Bakariya, B., Thakur, G.S.: Mining rare itemsets from weblog data. Natl. Acad. Sci. Lett. **39**, 359–363 (2016)

Improved CFDP Algorithms Based on Shared Nearest Neighbors and Transitive Closure

Li Ni, Wenjian Luo[(⊠)], Chenyang Bu, and Yamin Hu

Anhui Province Key Laboratory of Software Engineering in Computing
and Communication, School of Computer Science and Technology,
University of Science and Technology of China, Hefei 230027, Anhui, China
{nlcs,bucy1991,huym}@mail.ustc.edu.cn,
wjluo@ustc.edu.cn

Abstract. A recently proposed clustering algorithm named Clustering by fast search and Find of Density Peaks (CFDP) can automatically identify the cluster centers without an iterative process. The key step in CFDP is searching for the nearest neighbor with higher density for each point. However, the CFDP algorithm may not be effective for cases in which there exist density fluctuations within a cluster or between two nearby clusters. In this study, two improved algorithms named CFDP-ED-TSNN1 and CFDP-ED-TSNN2 are presented, which adopt different ways to utilize the dissimilarity. Here, the dissimilarity is based on shared nearest neighbors and transitive closure. The experimental results on both several artificial datasets and a real-world dataset show that the improved algorithms are competitive.

Keywords: Clustering · Shared nearest neighbors · Transitive closure

1 Introduction

Clustering aims to divide data points into different clusters according to the similarity between data points, ensuring that the data points in the same cluster have high similarity whereas data points in different clusters have low similarity [1–4]. Clustering has been extensively employed in various fields as an unsupervised machine learning method, such as community discovery [5]. Each clustering approach has its own advantages and disadvantages in different situations. It is generally known that k-Means [2] is simple and effective, but it is unable to handle clusters with non-spherical shapes and the number of clusters must be specified beforehand. DBSCAN [1], a representative density-based clustering algorithm, can find clusters with arbitrary shapes and does not need to know the number of clusters in advance. However, proper parameters should be determined. Moreover, it faces difficulties in handling clusters with significant differences in density.

Recently, in [6], Rodriguez and Laio proposed a novel clustering algorithm named CFDP. CFDP can automatically identify the cluster centers without an iterative process. However, the CFDP algorithm may not be effective for some cases, in which density fluctuations exist within a cluster or between two nearby clusters, such as those listed below.

U Kang et al. (Eds.): PAKDD 2017 Workshops, LNAI 10526, pp. 79–93, 2017.
DOI: 10.1007/978-3-319-67274-8_8

(1) When two local density maxima within a cluster are far away from each other, the CFDP might cluster these points into two clusters.

(2) When two local density maxima in different clusters are at a relatively small distance, the CFDP might cluster these points into one cluster.

(3) When a sparse cluster approaches a dense cluster, the sparse cluster may be clustered into the dense cluster by CFDP, because, the Most Similar Neighbor with Higher Density (MSNHD) in terms of Euclidean distance of a border point in the sparse cluster approaching the dense cluster, could be a point in the dense cluster.

In these cases, it seems that, if the dissimilarity based on Transitive closure and Shared Nearest Neighbors (TSNN) is used to find the MSNHD, the clustering results would be better. We call this method as CFDP-TSNN. However, experimental results demonstrate that the CFDP-TSNN still has its disadvantages.

Thus two improved algorithms named CFDP-ED-TSNN1 and CFDP-ED-TSNN2 are presented. The basic idea of CFDP-ED-TSNN1 is to cluster the data using CFDP first, and then adopts dissimilarity to identify and handle the clusters that were mistakenly clustered. The idea of CFDP-ED-TSNN2 is to reduce the cases mentioned above by adopting a combination of dissimilarity and distance to find the MSNHD. The comparisons between the improved algorithms and seven typical algorithms using both artificial datasets and a real-world dataset show that our algorithms are competitive.

The rest of this paper is organized as follows. The CFDP and dissimilarity are introduced in Sect. 2. The improved algorithms are described in Sect. 3. The experimental results are presented in Sect. 4. Section 5 concludes this paper briefly.

2   Related Work

2.1   CFDP Algorithm

Two assumptions are made in the CFDP [6], which are given as follows: (1) A cluster center is a local density maximum surrounded by their lower-density neighbors. (2) The distance between a cluster center and its MSNHD is large.

Here, the density of point i is computed by a Gaussian kernel [3], which is given as follows.

$$\rho_i = \sum_j exp\left(-\frac{d_{ij}^2}{d_c^2}\right) \tag{1}$$

where d_{ij} is the distance between points i and j, and d_c is the cutoff distance, which can be calculated using Eq. 2 [3].

$$d_c = distance\left[ceil\left(\frac{n*(n-1)}{2} * dc\_percent\right)\right] \tag{2}$$

where n is the size of the dataset; *dc_percent* is in the range [0.009, 0.045], function *ceil(x)* rounds x to the nearest integer greater than or equal to x, and *distance* is a vector storing the distance between all pairwise points in ascending order.

The distance between a point i and its MSNHD (i.e., δ_i) is the minimum distance between the point i and any other point with higher density (Eq. 3) [6]. The δ_i of point i with the highest density is set to the maximum distance between all pairwise points (i.e., Eq. 4), because the point does not have a MSNHD.

$$\delta_i = \min_{j:\rho_j > \rho_i} d_{ij} \tag{3}$$

$$\delta_i = \max_j \left(d_{ij} \right) \tag{4}$$

It can be easily seen that the value of δ_i of a local or global density maximum tends to be greater. Thus, a cluster center i can be characterized by a high ρ_i and a greater δ_i. According to this, the decision graph is adopted in [6] to identify the cluster centers. The horizontal axis of the graph represents ρ_i, and the vertical axis represents δ_i. Thus, the cluster centers are in the upper right region of the graph, and a gap is expected to exist between cluster centers and other points. Therefore, a parameter *threshold* can be manually set according to the decision graph to identify the cluster centers. Then, each of the rest points is allocated to the cluster that its MSNHD belongs to. For more details, please refer to reference [6].

2.2   TSNN Dissimilarity

2.2.1   Shared Nearest Neighbors

The similarity measure proposed by Jarvis and Patrick [7], is based on the shared nearest neighbors. Let $N_k(i)$ be the k-nearest neighbors of the point i. If both $i \in N_k(j)$ and $j \in N_k(i)$ are satisfied, the similarity between points i and j (denoted as sim_{ij}) can be calculated from Eq. 5, otherwise the value is 0.

$$sim_{ij} = \frac{N_k(i) \cap N_k(j)}{k} \tag{5}$$

Most elements in the similarity matrix $(sim_{ij})_{n*n}$ are zero, where n is the size of dataset. Only the similarity between a point and its k-nearest neighbors could be greater than 0. Besides, the similarity matrix is symmetrical.

This similarity measure can effectively distinguish the border points from different clusters. In the example shown in Fig. 1, points 6 and 9 are border points from different clusters. The two points can be clustered into one cluster by CFDP because they are close to each other. However, the two points can be clustered into different clusters correctly by adopting the above similarity measure. If $k = 5$, $N_5(6)$ are points 1, 2, 5, 6, and 7, and $N_5(9)$ are points 5, 6, 8, 10, and 11. The similarity between point 6 and point 9 is 0 because point 9 does not belong to $N_5(6)$. Thus, they are from different clusters.

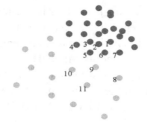

Fig. 1. Example of shared neighbors

2.2.2   Transitive Closure

The transitive closure algorithm proposed by Lee in [8] is adopted in this study to calculate the similarity between each pair of points. This algorithm is simple, and pseudo-code is given in Algorithm 1.

Algorithm 1:	An algorithm for computing the max-min transitive closure
Input:	The similarity matrix: $S = (sim_{ij})_{n*n}$
Output:	The max-min transitive closure of S: $B = (b_{ij})_{n*n}$
Step 1:	Elements in the B are set to -1
Step 2:	Construct a max heap for non-zero value elements in S
Step 3:	Set $b_{ii} = 1$, for $1 \le i \le n$
Step 4:	**While** there exists an element value of -1 in B and heap is not empty do
	Take top element s_{pq} of heap
	If b_{pq} is not -1, then calculate the following sets I and I' then
	Specifically, $I = \{j \mid b_{pj} \text{ is not } - 1\}$, $I' = \{i \mid b_{iq} \text{ is not } - 1\}$
	Set $b_{ij} = b_{ji} = s_{pq}$ where $i \in I$ and $j \in I'$
	End If
	Delete top element s_{pq} of heap
	End While
Step 5:	Set elements whose value is -1 to 0

The input matrix of Algorithm 1 is the similarity matrix $(sim_{ij})_{n*n}$ introduced in Sect. 2.2.1, which is based on the shared nearest neighbors. Therefore, the output matrix B of Algorithm 1 could represent the similarity of two points. Although the transitive closure based on shared neighbors in [9] is used for network data, whereas in this study, it is adopted to improve the CFDP algorithm for cases in which the density fluctuations exist within a cluster or between two nearby clusters.

The dissimilarity matrix can be calculated according to the matrix B. Specifically, the dissimilarity between points i and j (i.e., $Dissimi_{ij}$) is calculated by formula (6). For convenience, this dissimilarity is called as the *TSNN dissimilarity* in this study.

$$Dissimi_{ij} = 1 - b_{ij} \qquad (6)$$

Similar to the definition of δ_i, the *TSNN* dissimilarity between a point i and its MSNHD, i.e., γ_i, is the minimum between the point i and the other points with higher density. For the point with the highest density, its *TSNN* dissimilarity is set to the maximum *TSNN* dissimilarity, i.e., 1.

$$\gamma_i = \min_{j:\rho_j > \rho_i} (Dissimi_{ij}) \qquad (7)$$

Here, ρ_j and ρ_i represent the density of points i and j, respectively.

3 The Proposed Algorithms

3.1 Motivation

In Sect. 1, we have introduced some cases where the CFDP could be ineffective. Here, we take an example to illustrate its shortcomings.

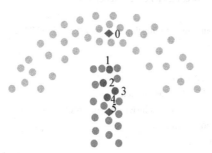

Fig. 2. An example of density fluctuations.

As shown in Fig. 2, point 1 would be falsely clustered into the cluster that point 0 belongs to. This is because point 0 is regarded as the MSNHD of point 1, rather than a point from the same cluster. Although point 5 is a point with greater density from the same cluster, the distance between point 5 and 1 is greater than the distance between point 0 and 1.

The use of *TSNN* dissimilarity, however, can correctly cluster the example shown in Fig. 2. The basic idea of adopting the *TSNN* dissimilarity is that points in the same cluster have small *TSNN* dissimilarity and points in different clusters have large *TSNN* dissimilarity. The *TSNN* dissimilarity between point 0 and 1 is 1 (no shared k-nearest neighbors), which is larger than the *TSNN* dissimilarity between point 5 and 1; thus, point 1 would be correctly assigned to the cluster that point 5 belongs to.

An intuition is to replace the Euclidean distance by the *TSNN* dissimilarity when we calculate the MSNHD of each point. The corresponding algorithm is named as CFDP-TSNN, and given in Algorithm 2, where the differences between CFDP-TSNN and CFDP are Steps 2, 7, and 8. However, the CFDP-TSNN also has some short-comings, especially when two clusters are adjacent. The disadvantages of the CFDP-TSNN will be demonstrated by experimental results (Sect. 4). That is to say, the CFDP-TSNN, which directly uses the TSNN dissimilarity to replace the Euclidean distance to calculate the MSNHD in the CFDP, is only used for experimental comparisons. Therefore in the rest of this Section, we present two algorithms, i.e., the CFDP-ED-TSNN1 and the CFDP-ED-TSNN2, to improve the performance of the CFDP.

Algorithm 2 :	CFDP-TSNN
Input:	Data set: D, Parameter: d_c
Output:	Clusters
Step 1:	Compute ρ_i (Eq. 1) and k-nearest neighbors for each point in D
Step 2:	Compute the TSNN dissimilarity matrix (see Section 2.2)
Step 3:	For each point i, compute γ_i (Eq. 7) and its MSNHD in terms of TSNN dissimilarity
Step 4:	Plot decision graph (γ_i as function of ρ_i) and determine the threshold [6]
Step 5:	Sort the data in descending order by density; recorded as $D1$
Step 6:	**For** each point i in $D1$ do
	If $\gamma_i >=threshold$ then
	Point i becomes a new cluster center
	Else:
	Assign point i to the cluster in which its MSNHD is contained
	End If
	End For
Step 7:	**For** each cluster $c \in C$ do
	If size of c is less than 4 then
	All points within cluster c are regarded as outliers
	Remove c from C
	End If
	End For
Step 8:	Sort outliers according to the density in descending order
	For each outlier point i do
	Assign point i to the cluster in which its MSNHD is contained
	End For

3.2   CFDP-ED-TSNN1

The basic idea of CFDP-ED-TSNN1 is given as follows. First, run CFDP to divide the points into several clusters. Then, adopt the TSNN dissimilarity to identify and handle the clusters that have been mistakenly clustered. Namely, if there exists two points in the same cluster, whose TSNN dissimilarity values are 1, it implies that at least two different clusters have been clustered into one group falsely. Thus, run CFDP-TSNN to divide these clusters correctly (see Step 4 in Algorithm 3). Moreover, for each two clusters c_1 and c_2, if both the average TSNN dissimilarity values of c_1 and c_2 are higher than the average *TSNN* dissimilarity value of the merged cluster of c_1 and c_2 (i.e., $c_1 \cup c_2$), it implies that c_1 and c_2 should be merged into one cluster (see Step 5 in Algorithm 3). The average *TSNN* dissimilarity value of a cluster c, i.e., $averageDis(c)$ is calculated using Eq. 8. According to the analysis above, if both Eqs. 9 and 10 are satisfied, c_1 and c_2 should be merged.

Algorithm3:	CFDP-ED-TSNN1
Input:	Data set: D, Parameter: d_c
Output:	Clusters
Step 1:	Compute ρ_i (Eq. 1) and k-nearest neighbors for each point in D
Step 2:	Compute the *TSNN* dissimilarity matrix (Section 2.2)
Step 3:	Divide the dataset into several clusters using CFDP; clustering results recorded as C
Step 4:	**For** each cluster $c \epsilon C$ **do**
	If there exists two points whose *TSNN* dissimilarity equals to 1 **then**
	Remove c from C
	Cluster c using CFDP-TSNN(Conduct Alg.2 except Step 8, *threshold*=1)
	Update the clustering results
	End If
	End For
Step 5:	**For** any two clusters $c_1, c_2 \epsilon C$ **do**
	If inequalities (9) and (10) are satisfied **then**
	Merge c_1 and c_2
	End If
	End For
Step 6:	Sort outliers according to the density in descending order
	For each outlier point i **do**
	Assign point i to the cluster in which its MSNHD in terms of distance is contained
	End For

$$averageDis(c) = \frac{\sum_{i \in c} \sum_{j \in c, j \neq i} Dissimi_{ij}}{n * (n - 1)/2} \qquad (8)$$

$$averageDis(c_1) \geq averageDis(c_1 \cup c_2) \qquad (9)$$

$$averageDis(c_2) \geq averageDis(c_1 \cup c_2) \qquad (10)$$

3.3   CFDP-ED-TSNN2

The idea of CFDP-ED-TSNN2 is to combine the *TSNN* dissimilarity and distance to determine an MSNHD. First, sort the points according to the density in descending order. Second, for every point, find the MSNHD in terms of distance and the MSNHD in terms of *TSNN* dissimilarity. Third, in addition to the cluster centers identified by the decision graph (briefly introduced in Sect. 2.1 and see [6] for details), the points with their γ_i values equal to 1 should also be regarded as the cluster centers. This is because for the case that the γ_i of point i is 1, it is very likely that point i and its MSNHD are not in the same cluster. Finally, for other points, use Eq. 11 to determine which clusters these points should be assigned to.

Algorithm 4: CFDP-ED-TSNN2

Input:	Data set: D, Parameter: d_c
Output:	Clusters

Step 1: Compute ρ_i (Eq. 1) and k-nearest neighbors for each point in D

Step 2: Compute the *TSNN* dissimilarity matrix (Section 2.2)

Step 3: Compute δ_i (Eq. 3) and γ_i (Eq. 7) for each point
  and record MSNHD in terms of distance and MSNHD in terms of *TSNN* dissimilarity

Step 4: Plot decision graph (plot δ_i as function of ρ_i) and determine the threshold [3]

Step 5: Sort points in descending order by density; recorded as *D1*

Step 6: **For** each point i in *D1* do
  If $\delta_i >$ **threshold** or $\gamma_i = 1$ **then**
    Point i becomes a new cluster center
  Else:
    Assign point i to the cluster of its MSNHD by Eq. 11
  End If
  End For

Step 7: **For** each cluster $c \in C$ do
  If size of c less than 4 **then**
    All points within cluster c are regarded as outliers; Remove c from C
  End If
  End For

Step 8: Sort outliers according to the density in descending order
  For each outlier point i do
    Assign point i to the cluster of its MSNHD by Eq. 11
  End For

For convenience, the MSNHD in terms of distance and the MSNHD in terms of *TSNN* dissimilarity of point i are denoted as s and t, respectively. If point s and t belong to the same cluster, then point i is also assigned to that cluster. Otherwise, the scores of both point s and t, i.e., $score_i(s)$ and $score_i(t)$, are calculated using Eq. 11 to determine which cluster point i should be assigned to. A higher score implies a higher similarity with the point i. Thus, point i should be assigned to the point with a higher score.

$$score_i(j) = \left(1 - Dissimi_{ij}\right) * \left(1 - \frac{d_{ij}}{d_{is} + d_{it}}\right) * \left(1 - \frac{\rho_j - \rho_i}{\rho_s + \rho_t - \rho_i}\right) \quad (11)$$

where j is s or t; d_{ij} is the distance between point i and j; ρ_i is the density of point i; and $Dissimi_{ij}$ is the *TSNN* dissimilarity between point i and j. The basic idea of Eq. 11 is that the point that has a smaller *TSNN* dissimilarity or less distance or less density difference with point i is more similar to the point, and the two points are more likely to be in the same cluster.

4   Experiments

4.1   Experimental Setup

The improved algorithms are tested on both artificial datasets and the Olivetti face dataset [10] by using the metric adjusted Rand index (ARI) [11]. The artificial datasets include six well-known datasets [12]: *Compound, Spiral, D31, R15, Aggregation*, and *Flame*. These artificial datasets have different shapes and densities. The Olivetti face dataset has 400 images of 40 people: each individual has 10 images with different expressions. However, for comparisons, only first 100 images are used to test the algorithms, as in [12].

For the artificial datasets, the improved algorithms are compared with the original CFDP [6], the variant of CFDP (i.e., CFDP-TSNN in Sect. 3.1), three classical algorithms (k-Means [2], DBSCAN [1], and OPTICS [13]), and other two state-of-the-art algorithms (CLASP [14] and CLUB [12]). For the Olivetti face dataset, the improved algorithms are compared with the CFDP, CFDP-TSNN, and CLUB algorithms. The experimental results of the compared algorithms (except CFDP-TSNN) are obtained from reference [12]. For convenience, CFDP-ED-TSNN1, CFDP-ED-TSNN2, and CFDP-TSNN are denoted as TSNN1, TSNN2, and TSNN respectively, in both Tables 1 and 2.a>

Table 1. Parameters of CFDP-ED-TSNN1, CFDP-ED-TSNN2, and CFDP-TSNN.

	Input parameters: (*dc_percent, threshold*)						
	Aggregation	Compound	D31	Flame	R15	Spiral	Olivetti
TSNN1	(0.034, 1.8)	(0.018, 6.0)	(0.01, 1.3)	(0.036, 6.2)	(0.025, 0.57)	(0.025, 3.2)	(0.043, 0.12)
TSNN2	(0.019, 5.8)	(0.018, 6.2)	(0.0095, 1.4)	(0.030, 6.2)	(0.023, 0.7)	(0.025, 3.2)	(0.031, 0.12)
TSNN	(0.024, 0.6)	(0.018, 0.6)	(0.023, 0.14)	(0.029, 0.4)	(0.037, 0,3)	(0.025, 0.8)	(0.033, 0.5)

Table 1 shows the parameters of the variants of CFDP. Parameter k of Eq. 5 is set according to Eq. 12. The basic concept of this setup is as follows. First, select s points from the dataset at $n/2s, 3n/2s, ..., n-n/2s$. The parameter s is calculated according to Eq. 13. Next, for the i-th point selected, count the number of points within distance d_c, that is, $num(i, d_c)$. The parameter d_c is calculated using Eq. 2. Finally, the average number is assigned to k.

$$k = ceil(\frac{1}{s} * (\sum_{i=1}^{i=s} num(i, d_c))) \qquad (12)$$

$$s = ceil(dc\_percent * n) \qquad (13)$$

where $ceil(x)$ rounds x to the nearest integer greater than or equal to x and n is the total number of points in the dataset.

4.2   Artificial Datasets

Figure 3 and Table 2 show the comparisons over the artificial datasets. Figure 3 shows the real clusters of these datasets in the left-most column, and the other three columns show the clustering results of CFDP-ED-TSNN1, CFDP-ED-TSNN2, and CFDP-TSNN. The points assigned to the same cluster are represented using the same color, except that the cluster centers identified are in red.

For the *compound* dataset, Fig. 3(b)–(d) shows that CFDP-TSNN identifies the two clusters on the upper-left corner as one cluster. However, the improved algorithms identify these clusters correctly, except at one point. In addition, Table 2 shows that the improved algorithms and CLUB show the best performance for the *compound* dataset.

For the *Spiral* dataset, Table 2 shows that CFDP-ED-TSNN1, CFDP-ED-TSNN2, CFDP-TSNN, CLUB, CFDP, and DBSCAN are all able to correctly identify the structure of the clusters. However, k-Means, CLASP, and OPTICS obtain poor results.

For dataset *D31*, k-Means achieves the best performance, followed by CLUB. The improved algorithms outperform other algorithms.

For dataset *R15*, Table 2 shows that CFDP-ED-TSNN1, CFDP-ED-TSNN2, CFDP, and k-Means obtain the best performances. Figures 3(m)–(p) show that almost all the points are correctly assigned to the clusters.

For the Aggregation dataset, Table 2 shows that CFDP-ED-TSNN1, CLUB, and CFDP identify the cluster structure exactly. Figure 3(s) shows that, for CFDP-ED-TSNN2 only one point is wrongly assigned. However, as shown in Fig. 3(t), CFDP-TSNN incorrectly divides adjacent clusters into the same clusters.

Table 2. Comparisons of the artificial datasets using the metric ARI. The rank of each algorithm on each dataset is provided following its value of ARI.

Algorithms	Compound	Spiral	D31	R15	Aggregation	Flame	Sum of ranks
TSNN1	**0.9972/1**	**1.0000/1**	0.9370/4	**0.9928/1**	**1.0000/1**	**1.0000/1**	9
TSNN2	**0.9972/1**	**1.0000/1**	0.9384/3	**0.9928/1**	0.9978/4	**1.0000/1**	11
TSNN	0.9438/4	**1.0000/1**	0.9227/6	0.9785/6	0.8089/8	0.9666/5	30
CLUB	**0.9972/1**	**1.0000/1**	0.9392/2	0.9910/5	**1.0000/1**	**1.0000/1**	11
CLASP	0.8173/7	0.0332/8	0.8781/7	0.6388/9	0.8580/6	0.0413/9	46
k-Means	0.5364/9	0.0058/9	**0.9523/1**	**0.9928/1**	0.7588/9	0.4112/8	37
DBSCAN	0.9078/6	**1.0000/1**	0.7406/9	0.9160/8	0.8539/7	0.8574/7	38
CFDP	0.5922/8	**1.0000/1**	0.9345/5	**0.9928/1**	**1.0000/1**	0.9881/4	20
OPTICS	0.9232/5	0.3075/7	0.8753/8	0.9600/7	0.9938/5	0.8962/6	38

For the Flame dataset, Table 2 shows that only CFDP-ED-TSNN1, CFDP-ED-TSNN2, and CLUB correctly identify the structure of the clusters.

The sum of all the ranks is shown in the right-most column of Table 2. The results show that CFDP-ED-TSNN1 outperforms all the algorithms, followed by CFDP-ED-TSNN2 and CLUB.

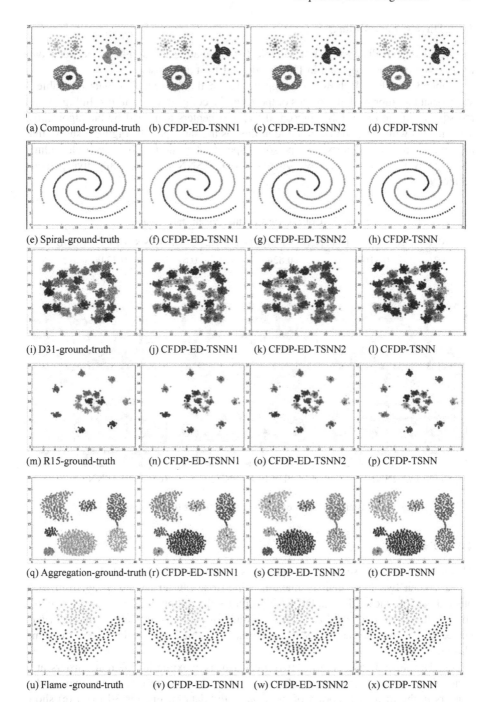

(a) Compound-ground-truth   (b) CFDP-ED-TSNN1   (c) CFDP-ED-TSNN2   (d) CFDP-TSNN

(e) Spiral-ground-truth   (f) CFDP-ED-TSNN1   (g) CFDP-ED-TSNN2   (h) CFDP-TSNN

(i) D31-ground-truth   (j) CFDP-ED-TSNN1   (k) CFDP-ED-TSNN2   (l) CFDP-TSNN

(m) R15-ground-truth   (n) CFDP-ED-TSNN1   (o) CFDP-ED-TSNN2   (p) CFDP-TSNN

(q) Aggregation-ground-truth (r) CFDP-ED-TSNN1   (s) CFDP-ED-TSNN2   (t) CFDP-TSNN

(u) Flame -ground-truth   (v) CFDP-ED-TSNN1   (w) CFDP-ED-TSNN2   (x) CFDP-TSNN

Fig. 3. Clustering results of improved algorithms and CFDP-TSNN on six datasets (Color figure online)

4.3   Olivetti Face Dataset

As the Euclidean distance is not suitable for calculating the similarity between two images, the method proposed in [15] is adopted for this dataset.

Table 3 and Fig. 4 show the comparisons on the Olivetti face dataset. Table 3 shows that the improved algorithms outperform the compared algorithms. In Fig. 4, the red squares in the upper left represent the cluster centers identified by the algorithms. The pictures with the same color are identified as the same people. Figure 4 shows that all three approaches identify nine persons. Specifically, the two improved algorithms identify seven persons correctly, whereas CFDP-TSNN identifies only five persons correctly.

Table 3. Comparisons on the Olivetti face dataset

Algorithms	CFDP-ED-TSNN1	CFDP-ED-TSNN2	CFDP-TSNN	CFDP	CLUB
ARI	0.8169	**0.8263**	0.6214	0.3244	0.7758

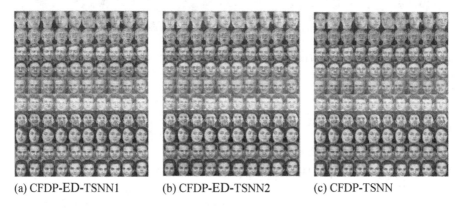

(a) CFDP-ED-TSNN1   (b) CFDP-ED-TSNN2   (c) CFDP-TSNN

Fig. 4. Clustering results of Olivetti face dataset (Color figure online)

4.4   Discussion

This subsection discusses the cases previously mentioned in the Sect. 1.

(1) When two local density maxima within one cluster are far away from each other, Fig. 5(a) shows that CFDP falsely divides the bottom cluster. Figures 5(b)–(d) show that the variants based on TSNN dissimilarity are able to identify these clusters correctly. This is because the TSNN dissimilarity is small when points are in the same cluster.

(2) The second case involves two local density maxima in different clusters at a relatively small distance to each other, as explained by the results on the two nearby clusters in the lower left corner of the *Compound* dataset. Figures 3(b) and (c) show that the improved algorithms are able to identify the two nearby clusters. However, the clustering result of CFDP (shown in Fig. 2(h) of [12]) shows that the inner cluster is

mistakenly clustered into the right-hand cluster. This is because the local density point of the inner cluster is very close to the local density point of the right-hand cluster; thus, the distance-based CFDP cannot distinguish the two clusters. However, the *TSNN* dissimilarity between the two points from the two disconnected clusters is 1, regardless of their proximity. Thus, the *TSNN* dissimilarity-based algorithms show good performance.

(3) The upper right corner of the Compound dataset shows when a sparse cluster nears a dense cluster. The clustering result of CFDP (shown in Fig. 2(h) of [12]) shows that two clusters are incorrectly identified as one cluster. However, Figs. 3(b) and (c) show that CFDP-ED-TSNN1 and CFDP-ED-TSNN2 successfully distinguish the sparse and dense clusters. This is because the TSNN dissimilarity is calculated based on the shared neighbors. As shown in Fig. 1 (analyzed in Sect. 2.2.1), the k-nearest neighbors of the border points of the dense cluster typically do not contain the points from the sparse cluster. Thus, the similarity between the border points of the dense and sparse clusters is zero. Accordingly, their *TSNN* dissimilarity values are 1. As a result, the two clusters can be distinguished.

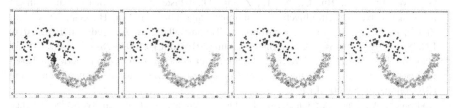

(a) CFDP (0.12, 6.6)   (b) TSNN1 (0.023, 14) (c) TSNN2 (0.019, 14)   (d)TSNN(0.02, 0.9)

Fig. 5. Clustering results on the dataset *Jain* [16]. The numbers in the parentheses are *dc_percent* and *threshold*. The red points are the identified cluster centers. (Color figure online)

(4) Table 2 shows that both CFDP-ED-TSNN1 and CFDP-ED-TSNN2 are better than CFDP-TSNN in most case, except the *Spiral* dataset where they have the same values of ARI. This demonstrates that CFDP-TSNN has poor clustering quality in some cases when, however, CFDP-ED-TSNN1 and CFDP-ED-TSNN2 obtain good clustering results.

5 Conclusions

In this study, we improved the CFDP algorithm for the cases in which the density fluctuations exist within a cluster or between two nearby clusters. Specifically, we presented two improved algorithms named CFDP-ED-TSNN1 and CFDP-ED-TSNN2. The first one is to cluster the data using CFDP first, and then adopts *TSNN* dissimilarity to identify and handle the clusters that were mistakenly clustered. The latter is to reduce the cases mentioned above by adopting a combination of *TSNN* dissimilarity and distance to find the MSNHD. Here, the *TSNN* dissimilarity is computed by shared nearest neighbors and transitive closure. The experiments on both artificial datasets and the real-world dataset show that our algorithm outperforms the original CFDP and is competitive with other state-of-the-art algorithms.

Acknowledgements. This work is partly supported by the Anhui Provincial Natural Science Foundation (No. 1408085MKL07).

References

1. Ester, M., Kriegel, H.-P., Sander, J., Xu, X.: A density-based algorithm for discovering clusters in large spatial databases with noise. In: KDD, pp. 226–231. AAAI (1996)
2. MacQueen, J.: Some methods for classification and analysis of multivariate observations. In: Proceedings of the Fifth Berkeley Symposium on Mathematical Statistics and Probability, pp. 281–297. University of California Press (1967)
3. Yan, Z., Luo, W., Bu, C., Ni, L.: Clustering spatial data by the neighbors intersection and the density difference. In: Proceedings of the 3rd IEEE/ACM International Conference on Big Data Computing, Applications and Technologies, pp. 217–226. ACM (2016)
4. Gao, W., Luo, W., Bu, C., Ni, L., Zhang, D.: Clustering evolutionary data with an r-dominance based multi-objective evolutionary algorithm. In: Yin, H., Gao, Y., Li, B., Zhang, D., Yang, M., Li, Y., Klawonn, F., Tallón-Ballesteros, A.J. (eds.) IDEAL 2016. LNCS, vol. 9937, pp. 342–352. Springer, Cham (2016). doi:10.1007/978-3-319-46257-8_37
5. Gao, W., Luo, W., Bu, C.: Evolutionary community discovery in dynamic networks based on leader nodes. In: 2016 International Conference on Big Data and Smart Computing (BigComp), pp. 53–60. IEEE (2016)
6. Rodriguez, A., Laio, A.: Clustering by fast search and find of density peaks. Science **344**(6191), 1492–1496 (2014)
7. Jarvis, R.A., Patrick, E.A.: Clustering using a similarity measure based on shared near neighbors. IEEE Trans. Comput. **100**(11), 1025–1034 (1973)
8. Lee, H.-S.: An optimal algorithm for computing the max–min transitive closure of a fuzzy similarity matrix. Fuzzy Sets Syst. **123**(1), 129–136 (2001)
9. Sun, P.G., Gao, L., Han, S.S.: Identification of overlapping and non-overlapping community structure by fuzzy clustering in complex networks. Inf. Sci. **181**(6), 1060–1071 (2011)
10. Samaria, F.S., Harter, A.C.: Parameterisation of a stochastic model for human face identification. In: Proceedings of the Second IEEE Workshop on Applications of Computer Vision, pp. 138–142. IEEE (1994)
11. Vinh, N.X., Epps, J., Bailey, J.: Information theoretic measures for clusterings comparison: is a correction for chance necessary? In: Proceedings of the 26th Annual International Conference on Machine Learning, pp. 1073–1080. ACM (2009)
12. Chen, M., Li, L.J., Wang, B., Cheng, J.J., Pan, L.N., Chen, X.Y.: Effectively clustering by finding density backbone based-on kNN. Pattern Recogn. **60**, 486–498 (2016)
13. Ankerst, M., Breunig, M.M., Kriegel, H.-P., Sander, J.: OPTICS: ordering points to identify the clustering structure. In: ACM Sigmod Record, pp. 49–60. ACM (1999)
14. Huang, H., Gao, Y., Chiew, K., Chen, L., He, Q.: Towards effective and efficient mining of arbitrary shaped clusters. In: 2014 IEEE 30th International Conference on Data Engineering, pp. 28–39. IEEE (2014)

15. Sampat, M.P., Wang, Z., Gupta, S., Bovik, A.C., Markey, M.K.: Complex wavelet structural similarity: a new image similarity index. IEEE Trans. Image Process. **18**(11), 2385–2401 (2009)

16. Jain, Anil K., Law, M.H.C.: Data clustering: a user's dilemma. In: Pal, S.K., Bandyopadhyay, S., Biswas, S. (eds.) PReMI 2005. LNCS, vol. 3776, pp. 1–10. Springer, Heidelberg (2005). doi:10.1007/11590316_1

CNN-Based Sequence Labeling for Fine-Grained Opinion Mining of Microblogs

Jiajun Cheng[✉], Pei Li, Xin Zhang, Zhaoyun Ding, and Hui Wang

College of Information Systems and Management,
National University of Defense Technology,
Hunan, Changsha, People's Republic of China
{jiajun.cheng,peili,xinzhang,zyding,huiwang}@nudt.edu.cn

Abstract. Opinion mining on microblogs is of significance because microblogging websites have attracted many users to share their experiences and express their opinions on a variety of topics. However, conventional opinion mining methods focus mainly on sentiment of texts and ignore opinion target. This paper focuses on a fine-grained opinion mining task that jointly extract opinion target and corresponding sentiment by sequence labeling. We propose a convolutional neural network (CNN)-based sequence labeling method and apply it to fine-grained opinion mining of microblogs. We empirically evaluated neural networks with different filter length and depth and analyzed the boundary of contextual feature extraction for opinion mining of microblogs. The experimental results demonstrate that the proposed CNN-based methods are better than RNN-based methods in both effectiveness and efficiency.

Keywords: Opinion mining · Microblogs · Convolutional neural network · Sequence labeling

1 Introduction

Microblog websites, such as Twitter and Sina Weibo, have attracted a number of users to express their opinions on variety of topics, making it invaluable sources of public opinions. Many researchers have investigated how to capture microblog users' opinion on products, services and public figures.

Conventional opinion mining methods mainly focus on sentiment classification of microblogs [1–3], which assign a sentiment score or sentiment polarity to represent the opinion expressed in a microblog. However, sentiment classification-based opinion mining may not meet the demands of fine-grained opinion mining because it ignores opinion targets. Besides, It may encounter some problems when a message expresses different opinions to different targets or the sentiment to a target is not the same with the sentiment of the message. Therefore, this paper focus on a fine-grained opinion mining task, i.e., sentiment parsing, which aims to jointly extract opinion target and corresponding sentiment [4].

© Springer International Publishing AG 2017
U Kang et al. (Eds.): PAKDD 2017 Workshops, LNAI 10526, pp. 94–103, 2017.
DOI: 10.1007/978-3-319-67274-8_9

Sentiment parsing aims to extract all $\langle T, S \rangle$ tuples from microblogging messages, where T means a target and S is the sentiment to target T. Sentiment parsing needs to find out all targets and sentiments as well as determine their relationships. It has been tackled as a sequence labeling problem in previous work [4]. This approach views a microblog sentence as a sequence of tokens labeled with the "PNO" tagging scheme: P denotes that the token is inside an opinion target and the sentiment to the target is positive; N indicates a token inside an opinion target and the sentiment to the target is negative; and O is used for other tokens in the sentence. An example sentence and the corresponding labels are shown in Table 1, the labels denote that the sentence expresses positive sentiment to "Russell Westbrook" and negative sentiment to "Steph Curry".

Table 1. An example sentence with labels.

Sentence	I	think	Russell	Westbrook	plays	better	than	Steph	Curry
Label	O	O	P	P	O	O	O	N	N	O

Convolution neural network (CNN) is well known as its capability of capturing contextual information and has been successfully applied to variety of natural language processing tasks such as character-level word embedding [5–7], text classification [8–10], sentiment analysis [11,12], machine translation [13] and Web search [14]. However, because sequence length always decreases after CNN layers, CNN is rarely used in word-level sequence labeling tasks. This motivate us to propose a CNN-based sequence labeling method and explore an application of CNN to the task of sentiment parsing. To evaluate the proposed method, we compare it with RNN-based sequence labeling method and experimental results show that the proposed method is better than RNN-based sequence labeling method in both effectiveness and efficiency.

2   Related Works

Opinion mining of microblogs. Microblogging websites are invaluable sources of public opinions and many studies have been launched on opinion mining of microblogs. Early studies on opinion mining of microblogs usually build a sentiment lexicon and calculate a sentiment score for each microblog message. O'Connor et al. [15] calculate a sentiment score for each tweet and summarize the scores of tweets containing the candidates to predict the approval ratings in elections. Bollen et al. [1] use a sentiment lexicon to determine the ratio of positive versus negative tweets on a given day and apply it in the stock market predicting. Some learning-based approach are applied to opinion mining of microblogs. Kumaresan [2] propose a hybrid architecture for twitter sentiment classification by combining random forest, SVM and naive Bayesian classifier. Hu [3] takes social relation into consideration and determines sentiment of tweets with the text and social relations of the user. Bravo [16] combines strengths, emotions and polarities for sentiment analysis of twitter. However, these studies focus mainly on sentiment of microblogs and ignores opinion target. Therefore, we defined a fine-grained opinion mining task, i.e., sentiment parsing, of microblogs and applied RNN to the task in previous work [4]. This paper focuses on sentiment parsing task as well and attempts to improve the performance of sequence labeling.

CNN in NLP. Owing to the capability of capturing local correlations of spatial or temporal structures, CNNs have been successfully applied to many NLP tasks. Some studies prove that CNN is an effective approach to grasp morphological information and apply it to generate word embedding in character-level [5–7]. They combine conventional word-level embedding, character-level embedding generated by CNN and additional word-level features to construct features of each word and use these features as input of high level neural networks for different NLP tasks. In word-level processing, a lot of researches employ CNN for text modeling and further exploit the text features in document-level and sentence-level NLP tasks, such as text classification [8–10], sentiment analysis [11,12], machine translation [13] and Web search [14]. However, because the dimension of features always decrease sharply through CNN layers, only a few work utilizes CNNs for sequence labeling in NLP. Xu et al. [17] use a CNN layer to learn word features in window context and employ a TriCRF layer for slot filling and intent detection. The model achieves the stat-of-the-art in both tasks. Therefore, this paper attempts to apply CNN to sequence labeling problem for sentiment parsing of microblogs.

3   Methodology

This section introduces the neural network architecture and explains how to extract opinion target and sentiment polarity jointly with CNN based sequence labeling. As show in Fig. 1, the neural network architecture contains three kinds of layers: embedding layer projects word into fixed-length vectors; convolution layers extract features of each word in sentence; labeling layer predicts label of each word with the features from convolution layers.

3.1   Word Embedding

Word embedding layer aims to represent each word with a vector and thus words can be calculated in high-level layers. Bengio et al. [18] suggest that learning jointly the representation (word embedding) and language model is very useful. Collobert et al. [19] point out that pre-trained word embedding on large unlabeled datasets are useful for different tasks, and they released their word embedding trained on Wikipedia. Recent years, word embedding is commonly used in most of neural network-based natural language processing tasks. Different training models for word embedding, such as Word2Vec [20] and Glove [21],

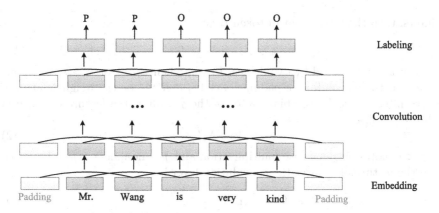

Fig. 1. An illustration of CNN-based sequence labeling for sentiment parsing task.

are proposed. Specifically, let D represents the token dictionary of a dataset, word embedding $E \in R^{d \times |D|}$ represents each token $t \in D$ with a fixed-length vector $e_t \in R^d$. The embedding matrix E is usually pre-trained with a large unsupervised dataset and taken as a group of parameters in task-specific training process. Lai et al. [22] analyzed different corpus and different embedding models, pointing out that corpus domain is more important than corpus size. Therefore, this paper trains word embedding on a microblog corpus with Word2Vec [20].

3.2 Convolution

In sentiment parsing task, the label of a word in a sentence is determined by the meaning of the word as well as its contextual information. Word embedding layer expresses general meaning of each word with a vector, and convolution layer aims to extract contextual information of each word.

Generally, CNN has two kinds of operations, i.e., convolution and pooling. Convolution operation extracts steady contextual features by sliding some fixed-length windows. Each window, usually called a filter, extract one type of contextual feature in different locations with the same weights. Pooling operation aggregate features over a region by calculating the maximum or mean value of the features in the region. Multi-layers of alternate convolution and pooling operations can extract features in different scales. For sequence labeling tasks, the length of output sequence usually needs to be same with input sequence. However, both convolution and pooling will reduce the dimension of sequence, making it rarely used in sequence labeling tasks. In order to keep the length of sequence, this paper discard pooling operation, because it reduces sequence length sharply, and add some paddings to the beginning and end of sentences according to filter size and number of layers.

For a sentence $S = \{t_1, t_2, ..., t_s\}$, each token t_i has been projected to be a vector e_{t_i}. In a convolution layer, suppose m is the filter length, n is the number of filters, then the filter input of token t_i is:

$$X_i = [e_{t_{i-m/2+1/2}}, ..., e_{t_i}, ... e_{t_{i+m/2-1/2}}], \tag{1}$$

where m is set to be odd to void bias. In X_i, when $k < 1$ or $k > s$, $e_{t_k} = e_p$, where e_p is the embedding of padding. Let $W_j \in R^{m \times d}$ be the weight matrix of the jth filter and b_j be the bias vector of the jth filter, the feature of token t_j with the jth filter is:

$$c_{ij} = f(W_j \circ X_i^T + b_j), \tag{2}$$

where $\circ$ denotes element-wise multiplication and f is nonlinear active function. Then the feature of t_j after the convolution layer is

$$C_i = [c_{i1}, c_{i2}, ..., c_{in}]^T. \tag{3}$$

For multilayer of convolution, we use same filter length in one model for different layers. We define CWS as the covered window size, which represents the number of tokens covered by CNN layers when determine the label of a token. For example, in one convolution layer with filter length m, the covered window of token t_i is $[t_{i-m/2+1/2}, ..., t_i, ..., t_{i+m/2-1/2}]$ and the covered window size is m, which means that the label of t_i is only determined by the m tokens around it (including itself). When depth of convolution layer increase, each layer will add $(m-1)$ tokens into the covered window. Therefore, the covered window size is determined by filter length m and depth dep of convolution layer:

$$CWS(m, dep) = m + (m-1) * (dep - 1) = (m - 1) * dep + 1. \tag{4}$$

Covered window size determines the boundary of contextual feature extraction and thus is a significant indicator of the capability of a model.

3.3   Labeling

As mentioned before, we use the "PNO" tagging scheme to formulate sentiment parsing to be a sequence labeling problem in this paper. Let $L = \{l_1, l_2, ..., l_s\}$ denotes the label sequence of sentence $S = \{t_1, t_2, ..., t_s\}$, where $l_i \in \{P, N, O\}$ is the label of t_i. In labeling layer, We represent each label with a normalized 3-dimensional vector. For instance, the label vector is of token t_i is

$$\hat{y}_i = \begin{cases} (1, 0, 0), & where \ l_i = P \\ (0, 1, 0), & where \ l_i = N \\ (0, 0, 1), & where \ l_i = O \end{cases} \tag{5}$$

Labeling layer translates the output of convolution layer at each step into a three-dimension vector and normalize it with a softmax function:

$$y_i = softmax(WC_i + b), \tag{6}$$

where W is a weight matrix and b is a bias vector. The summation of elements in y_i is 1 and each element in y_j can be seen as the probability of its related label. For instance, vector $(0.6, 0.3, 0.1)$ denotes that the label of the corresponding token has the probability of 0.6 to be P, 0.3 to be N, and 0.1 to be O.

3.4   Training and Prediction

In training process, $\theta = \{E, W_*, b_*\}$ is the set of model parameters. Neural network predicts a label code y_i for each token t_i in each sentence, we take the cross-entry error of y_i and $\hat{y}_i$ as the loss of token t_i:

$$L_{ce}(\hat{y}_i, y_i; \theta) = -\sum_{k=0}^{2} \hat{y}_{ik} \log y_{ik}. \tag{7}$$

The loss value of training dataset is the mean loss value of all tokens in training dataset:

$$L(\theta) = \frac{1}{N} \sum_{i=1}^{N} \frac{1}{s_j} \sum_{i=1}^{s_j} L_{ce}(\hat{y}_i, y_i; \theta). \tag{8}$$

where N is the number of sentences in training dataset.

In predicting process, each token in a sentence get a label code through the neural network. The largest element in the output vectors represents the predicted label of this token in the sentence.

4   Experiment

4.1   Experiment Setting

We evaluate the proposed CNN-based method on a Chinese microblog dataset [4], which is collected from Sina Weibo and contains messages and replies of 5 controversial hot topics. The dataset have 67,033 unlabeled messages and 5000 labeled sentences. Each labeled message have been annotated with the mentioned targets and corresponding sentiment. We train word embedding on the 67,033 unlabeled messages with Word2Vec [20] and take it as initial word embedding. We use F-score of opinion tuples in labeled messages and training time to evaluate the effectiveness and efficiency of different models, respectively.

RNN-based sequence labeling method is taken as the baseline. Specifically, according to the experiment of previous work [4], we compare the proposed method with bidirectional simple RNN(SRNN), long short term memory(LSTM) and gated recurrent unit(GRU) at depth from 1 to 5. We explore four different filter lengths (3, 5, 7 and 9) with seven different convolutions layers (from 1 to 7) and compare the F-score and training time with RNN-based methods. All models are trained via the Adam optimizer [23]. We implement the neural networks using the Keras library[1], a highly modular neural networks library. The models are running on a NVIDIA GeForce GTX1080 GPU.

---

[1] https://github.com/fchollet/keras.

4.2 Result and Discussion

Effectiveness. The F-scores of different models are displayed in Fig. 2, different lines represent different models and each line is the F-scores in different layers. The solid lines are CNN-based methods and dashed lines are RNN-based methods. When the depth increase, F-scores of all models increase at first and tend to decrease after a depth. However, CNN-based methods are steadier than RNN-based methods because their F-score does not decrease sharply after reaching the best depth. Most CNN-based models achieve better result than RNN-based methods. CNN-based models with filter length 5 and 7 are better than models with filter length 3 and 9. The best F-score is 0.631, achieved by CNN-based method of two convolution layers with filer length 7. It is better than the best F-score of RNN-based method—0.622.

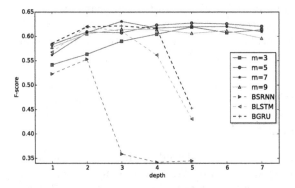

Fig. 2. F-score of different neural networks.

Efficiency. The training time of different models are shown in Fig. 3 and the setting of lines are same with Fig. 2. It can be seen that the time cost of CNN-based methods are much less than that of RNN-based methods. When neural network layers increase, the time cost of RNN-based methods increases linearly and that of RNN-based methods increase exponentially. Besides, from the detail figure of CNN-based methods in the upper-left corner, it can be seen that the training time of CNN-based methods is mainly determined by number of CNN layers. When filter length increase, the training time increases slightly.

Covered window size. In order to find the relationship of performance and covered window size, we calculate the covered window size of each neural network and compare it with the length distribution of sentence and sub-sentence in the dataset. As show in Fig. 4, the sub-figure at the top is F-scores of neural networks in different covered window sizes. When covered window extends, performance of neural networks become better at first and keep steady after that. When covered window size is larger than 10, the performance tends to keep steady.

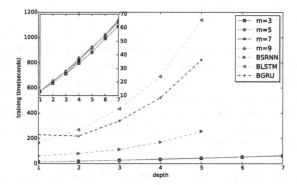

Fig. 3. Training time of different neural networks. The sub-figure in the upper-left corner is details of training time of CNN-based methods.

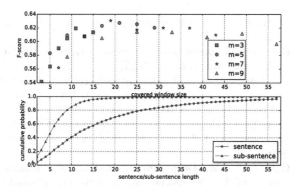

Fig. 4. Performance of CNN-based methods in different covered window size. The sub-figure at the top is F-scores of neural networks in different covered window size. The sub-figure at the bottom is the cumulative probability distribution of the length of sentences and sub-sentences in the dataset.

When covered window size is near 20, neural networks get best performance and begin to get worse. The sub-figure at the bottom is the cumulative probability distribution of the length of sentences and sub-sentences in the dataset. 85% of sub-sentences are short than 10 tokens and 98% of sub-sentences are short than 20 tokens. Therefore, neural networks with covered window size 10 cover most of sub-sentences when determine the label of a token; and neural networks with covered window size 20 cover most of sub-sentences and their neighboring sub-sentences when determine the label of a token. This indicates that most opinions may not be expressed in a sub-sentences. When we wish to extract opinion accurately, we should consider more than one sub-sentence for an opinion.

5   Conclusion

In this paper, we focus on a fine-grained sentiment analysis task—sentiment parsing—of microblogs. We propose a CNN-based sequence labeling method and apply it to sentiment parsing task. We empirically evaluated neural networks with different filter length and depth and analyzed the influence of covered window size of CNN neural networks to opinion mining of microblogs. Experiments show that the proposed CNN-based methods perform better than RNN-based sequence labeling in both effectiveness and efficiency.

Acknowledgments. The research is supported by National Natural Science Foundation of China (No. 71331008).

References

1. Bollen, J., Mao, H., Zeng, X.: Twitter mood predicts the stock market. J. Comput. Sci. **2**(1), 1–8 (2011)
2. Kumaresan, R.: A hybrid approach for supervised twitter sentiment classification. Int. J. Comput. Sci. Bus. Inf. **7**(1), 35 (2013)
3. Hu, X., Tang, L., Tang, J., Liu, H.: Exploiting social relations for sentiment analysis in microblogging. In: Proceedings of the Sixth ACM International Conference on Web Search and Data Mining, pp. 537–546. ACM (2013)
4. Cheng, J., Zhang, X., Li, P., Zhang, S., Ding, Z., Wang, H.: Exploring sentiment parsing of microblogging texts for opinion polling on Chinese public figures. Appl. Intell. 1–14 (2016)
5. dos Santos, C.N., Gatti, M.: Deep convolutional neural networks for sentiment analysis of short texts. In: Proceedings of the 25th International Conference on Computational Linguistics (COLING), Dublin, Ireland (2014)
6. Chiu, J.P.C., Nichols, E.: Named entity recognition with bidirectional lstm-cnns. arXiv preprint arXiv:1511.08308 (2015)
7. Ma, X., Hovy, E.: End-to-end sequence labeling via bi-directional lstm-cnns-crf. arXiv preprint arXiv:1603.01354 (2016)
8. Kim, Y.: Convolutional neural networks for sentence classification. arXiv preprint arXiv:1408.5882 (2014)
9. Johnson, R., Zhang, T.: Effective use of word order for text categorization with convolutional neural networks. arXiv preprint arXiv:1412.1058 (2014)
10. Lai, S., Xu, L., Liu, K., Zhao, J.: Recurrent convolutional neural networks for text classification. In: Twenty-Ninth AAAI Conference on Artificial Intelligence (2015)
11. Wu, H., Gu, Y., Sun, S., Gu, X.: Aspect-based opinion summarization with convolutional neural networks. arXiv preprint arXiv:1511.09128 (2015)
12. Tang, D., Qin, B., Liu, T.: Document modeling with gated recurrent neural network for sentiment classification. In: Proceedings of the 2015 Conference on Empirical Methods in Natural Language Processing, pp. 1422–1432 (2015)
13. Meng, F., Lu, Z., Wang, M., Li, H., Jiang, W., Liu, Q.: Encoding source language with convolutional neural network for machine translation. arXiv preprint arXiv:1503.01838 (2015)

14. Shen, Y., He, X., Gao, J., Deng, L., Mesnil, G.: Learning semantic representations using convolutional neural networks for web search. In: Proceedings of the Companion Publication of the 23rd International Conference on World Wide Web Companion, pp. 373–374. International World Wide Web Conferences Steering Committee (2014)

15. O'Connor, B., Balasubramanyan, R., Routledge, B.R., Smith, N.A.: From tweets to polls: linking text sentiment to public opinion time series. ICWSM **11**(122–129), 1–2 (2010)

16. Bravo-Marquez, F., Mendoza, M., Poblete, B.: Combining strengths, emotions and polarities for boosting twitter sentiment analysis. In: Proceedings of the Second International Workshop on Issues of Sentiment Discovery and Opinion Mining, p. 2. ACM (2013)

17. Xu, P., Sarikaya, R.: Joint intent detection and slot filling using convolutional neural networks. In: Proceedings of the IEEE International Conference on Acoustics, Speech, and Signal Processing (2014)

18. Bengio, Y., Schwenk, H., Senécal, J.S., Morin, F., Gauvain, J.L.: Neural probabilistic language models. In: Holmes, D.E., Jain, L.C. (eds.) Innovations in Machine Learning. Studies in Fuzziness and Soft Computing, vol. 194. Springer, Berlin (2006). doi:10.1007/3-540-33486-6_6

19. Collobert, R., Weston, J., Bottou, L., Karlen, M., Kavukcuoglu, K., Kuksa, P.: Natural language processing (almost) from scratch. J. Mach. Learn. Res. **12**, 2493–2537 (2011)

20. Mikolov, T., Sutskever, I., Chen, K., Corrado, G., Dean, J.: Distributed representations of words and phrases and their compositionality. arXiv preprint arXiv:1310.4546 (2013)

21. Pennington, J., Socher, R., Manning, C.D.: Glove: global vectors for word representation. In: Proceedings of the Empiricial Methods in Natural Language Processing (EMNLP 2014), vol. 12 (2014)

22. Lai, S., Liu, K., Xu, L., Zhao, J.: How to generate a good word embedding? arXiv preprint arXiv:1507.05523 (2015)

23. Kingma, D., Ba, J.: Adam: a method for stochastic optimization. arXiv preprint arXiv:1412.6980 (2014)

A Genetic Algorithm for Interpretable Model Extraction from Decision Tree Ensembles

Gilles Vandewiele[✉], Kiani Lannoye, Olivier Janssens, Femke Ongenae,
Filip De Turck, and Sofie Van Hoecke

Department of Information Technology,
Ghent University - imec, IDLab, Ghent, Belgium
{gilles.vandewiele,kiani.lannoye,olivier.janssens,
femke.ongenae,filip.deturck,sofie.vanhoecke}@ugent.be

Abstract. Models obtained by decision tree induction techniques excel in being interpretable. However, they can be prone to overfitting, which results in a low predictive performance. Ensemble techniques provide a solution to this problem, and are hence able to achieve higher accuracies. However, this comes at a cost of losing the excellent interpretability of the resulting model, making ensemble techniques impractical in applications where decision support, instead of decision making, is crucial.

To bridge this gap, we present the GENESIM algorithm that transforms an ensemble of decision trees into a single decision tree with an enhanced predictive performance while maintaining interpretability by using a genetic algorithm. We compared GENESIM to prevalent decision tree induction algorithms, ensemble techniques and a similar technique, called ISM, using twelve publicly available data sets. The results show that GENESIM achieves better predictive performance on most of these data sets compared to decision tree induction techniques & ISM. The results also show that GENESIM's predictive performance is in the same order of magnitude as the ensemble techniques. However, the resulting model of GENESIM outperforms the ensemble techniques regarding interpretability as it has a very low complexity.

Keywords: Decision support · Decision tree merging · Genetic algorithms

1 Introduction

Decision tree induction is a white-box machine learning technique that obtains an easily interpretable model after training. For each prediction from the model, an accompanying explanation can be given. Moreover, as opposed to rule extraction algorithms, the complete structure of the model is easy to analyze as it is encoded in a decision tree.

In domains where the decisions that need to be made are critical, the emphasis of machine learning is on offering support and advice to the experts instead

U Kang et al. (Eds.): PAKDD 2017 Workshops, LNAI 10526, pp. 104–115, 2017.
DOI: 10.1007/978-3-319-67274-8_10

of making the decisions for them. As such, the interpretability and comprehensibility of the obtained models are of primal importance for the experts that need to base their decision on them. Therefore, a white-box approach is preferred. Examples of critical domains include the medical domain (e.g. cardiology and oncology), the financial domain (e.g. claim management and risk assessment) and law enforcement.

One of the disadvantages of decision trees is that they are prone to overfit [1]. To overcome this shortcoming, ensemble techniques have been proposed. These techniques combine the results of different classifiers, leading to an improvement in the prediction performance because of three reasons [2]. First, when the amount of training data is small compared to the size of the hypothesis space, a learning algorithm can find many different hypotheses that correctly classify all the training data, while not performing well on unseen data. By averaging the results of the different hypotheses, the risk of choosing a wrong hypothesis can be reduced. Second, many learning algorithms can get stuck in local optima. By constructing different models from different starting points, the chance to find the global optimum is increased. Third, because of the finite size of the training data set, the optimal hypothesis can be outside of the space searched by the learning algorithm. By combining classifiers, the search space gets extended, again increasing the chance to find the optimal classifier. Nevertheless, ensemble techniques also have disadvantages. First, they take considerably longer to train and make a prediction. Second, their resulting models require more storage. The third and most important disadvantage is that the obtained model consists either out of many decision trees or only one decision tree that contains uninterpretable nodes (which is the case for stacking), making it infeasible or impossible for experts to interpret and comprehend the obtained model. To bridge the gap between decision tree induction algorithms and ensemble techniques, post-processing methods are required that can convert the ensemble into a single model. By first constructing an ensemble from the data and then applying this post-processing method, a better predictive performance can possibly be achieved compared to constructing a decision tree from the data directly.

This post-processing technique is not only useful to increase the predictive performance while maintaining excellent interpretability. It can also be used in a big data setting where an interpretable model is required and the size of the training data set is too large to construct a predictive model on a single node in a feasible amount of time. To solve this, the data set can be partitioned and a predictive model can be constructed for each of these partitions in a distributed fashion. Finally, the different models can be combined together.

In this paper, we present a novel post-processing technique for ensembles, called GENetic Extraction of a Single, Interpretable Model (GENESIM), which is able to convert the different models from the ensemble into a single, interpretable model. Since each of the models in the ensemble being merged will have an impact on the predictive performance of the final combined model, a genetic approach is applied which combines models from different subsets of an ensemble. The outline of the rest of this paper is as follows. First, in Sect. 2, work related to genetic decision tree evolving and decision tree merging is discussed. Then, in Sect. 3, the different steps of GENESIM are described. In Sect. 4, a comparison regarding predictive performance and model complexity is made between GENESIM, a similar technique called ISM and prevalent ensemble & decision tree induction techniques. Finally, in Sect. 5, a conclusion and possible future work are presented.

2   Related Work

In the work of Kargupta et al. [3], decision trees are merged by first converting them to the spectral domain using a Fourier transformation. Next, the obtained spectra of different trees are added together and the inverse Fourier transformation converts the spectrum back to a decision tree. Although promising, this method has not yet been applied successfully in any real-life application.

Quinlan proposed MiniBoosting [4], wherein three boosting iterations are applied and the small resulting decision trees are merged into one very large tree, which can finally be pruned to enhance generalization. This technique has a higher accuracy than a single decision tree for the largest part of twenty-seven tested data sets, but a lower accuracy than the boosting implementation ADABOOST.

A more straight-forward technique is proposed by Quinlan [5] which translates the decision trees in production rules that are much easier to simplify than the trees themselves. Next, the production rules are either represented as a decision table, or transformed in a set of k-dimensional hyperplanes, and subsequently merged using algorithms such as the MIL algorithm [6] or respectively by calculating the intersection of the hyperplanes [7].

In the work of Van Assche et al. [8], a technique called Interpretable Single Model (ISM) is proposed. This technique is very similar to an induction algorithm, as it constructs a decision tree recursively top-down, by first extracting a fixed set of possible candidate tests from the trees in the ensemble. For each of these candidate tests, a split criterion is calculated by estimating the parameters using information from the ensemble instead of the training data. Then, the test with the optimal split criterion is chosen and the algorithm continues recursively until a pre-prune condition is met. Two shortcomings of this approach can be identified. First, information from all models, including the ones that will have a negative impact, are used to construct a final model. Second, because of the similarity with induction algorithms, it is possible to get stuck in the same local optimum as these algorithms.

Deng [9] introduced STEL, which converts an ensemble into an ordered rule list using the following steps. First, for each tree in the ensemble, each path from the root to a leaf is converted into a classification rule. After all rules are extracted, they are pruned and ranked to create an ordered rule list. This sorted rule set can then be used for classification by iterating over each rule and returning the target when a matching rule is found. While a good predictive performance is reported for this technique, it is much harder to grasp an ordered rule list completely

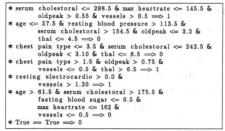

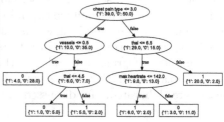

(a) The resulting model for STEL for one of the three folds for the heart disease data set.

(b) The resulting model for GENESIM for one of the three folds for the heart disease data set.

Fig. 1. Comparison of the resulting models of STEL and GENESIM regarding model complexity

than a decision tree, as can be seen in Fig. 1. Therefore, when interpretability is of primal importance, the post-processing technique, that converts the ensemble of models into a single model, should result in a decision tree.

It is impossible to know a priori which subset of decision trees should be merged to obtain the most accurate model. A brute-force approach that tries every possible combination would require an infeasible amount of computation time. Therefore, a genetic approach is applied that merges different decision trees for several iterations. Genetic (or evolutionary) algorithms are meta-heuristics most often used in optimization problems [10]. A recent and thorough survey of evolutionary algorithms for decision tree evolving can be found in [11].

3 GENESIM: GENetic Extraction of a Single, Interpretable Model

While in Barros et al. [11], genetic algorithms are discussed to construct decision trees from the data directly, in this paper, a genetic algorithm is applied on an ensemble of decision trees, created by using well-known induction algorithms combined with techniques such as bagging and boosting. Applying a genetic approach allows to efficiently traverse the very large search space of possible model combinations. This results in an innovative approach for merging decision trees which takes advantage of the positive properties of creating an ensemble. By exploiting multi-objective optimization, the resulting algorithm increases the accuracy ánd decreases the decision tree size at the same time, while most of the state-of-the-art succeeds in only one of the two.

A genetic algorithm generally consists of 6 phases, which are repeated iteratively. First, in an initialization phase, the population of candidate solutions is generated. It is important that the initial population is diverse enough, to allow for an extensive search space and reduce the chance of being stuck at local optima. Second, in each iteration, the individuals are evaluated using a fitness function. Then, in a selection phase, pairs of individuals are selected based on their fitness in order to combine them. In a fourth phase, the selected individuals are recombined, resulting in new offsprings. Furthermore, in each iteration, an individual has a certain probability to be mutated. Finally, in the end of each iteration, new offsprings are added to the population and the least fit individuals are discarded. In the subsequent subsections, each of the genetic algorithm phases are elaborated, and discussed in context of GENESIM[1].

3.1 Initialization Phase

First, the training data is divided into a new training set and a validation set. Then, different induction algorithms, including C4.5, CART, QUEST and GUIDE are applied on the training data in combination with bagging. Moreover, an ADABOOST classifier is trained and each of the decision trees of its resulting model is added to the population.

3.2 Evaluation Phase

The fitness function in GENESIM is defined to be the classification rate on the validation set:

$$accuracy = \frac{1}{N} * \sum_{1}^{N} \mathbb{1}_{g(x_i)=y_i}$$

with N the length of the validation data set and $g()$ the hypothesis of the individual. When two individuals have the same accuracy, the one with the lowest model complexity (expressed as number of nodes in the tree) is preferred.

3.3 Selection Phase

In each iteration, deterministic tournament selection is applied to select the individuals which will get recombined in the next phase. Tournament selection has two hyper-parameters: k and p. It chooses k individuals from the population at random and sorts them by their fitness. Then, the best individual from the tournament is returned with probability p, the second best individual with probability $p * (1 - p)$, the third best with probability $p * (1 - p)^2$, and so on. In deterministic tournament selection, p is equal to 1 and thus the best individual from the tournament is always returned.

3.4 Recombination Phase

To merge decision trees together, they are first converted to sets of k-dimensional hyperplanes (called the decision space), k being the number of features, by defining a unidirectional one-to-one mapping. Each node in a decision tree corresponds to a hyperplane in the decision space. Consequently, each leaf of the decision tree corresponds to a hyperrectangle in the decision space. An example of such a conversion can be seen in Fig. 2.

---

[1] https://github.com/IBCNServices/GENESIM.

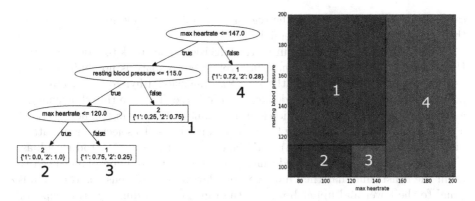

Fig. 2. Converting a decision tree to its set of k-dimensional hyperplanes. The decision tree is generated using C4.5, on the heart disease data set with two features: maximum heart rate and resting blood pressure. The color red in the decision space corresponds to class 1, the color blue corresponds to class 2. The purple tint, which consists out of a certain percentage of blue and red color, corresponds to the distribution of the two classes in a leaf. (Color figure online)

When all the nodes from all the trees are converted to their corresponding hyperplane, the different decision spaces can be merged together by calculating their intersection using a sweep line approach discussed in [7]. In this approach, each hyperplane is projected on a line segment in each dimension. These line segments are then sorted, making it easy to find the intersecting line segments in one specific dimension. In the end, if the projected line segments of two hyperplanes intersect in each dimension, the hyperplanes intersect as well. Subsequently, their intersection can be calculated and added to the resulting decision space. This method requires $O(k*n*log(n))$ computational time, with k the dimensionality of the data and n the number of planes in the sets, opposed to the quadratic complexity of a naive approach which calculates the intersection of each possible pair of planes.

The resulting decision spaces can contain many different regions as the number of regions in a merged space can increase quadratically in worst-case with the amount of regions in the original spaces. In order to reduce the amount of regions in the resulting space, and thus the amount of nodes in the merged decision tree (possibly leading to better generalization), the decision space should be pruned. Pruning can be achieved by combining two regions with similar class distributions (i.e. color in Fig. 2) that are next to each other. Similarity of class distributions can be measured by using a distance metric such as the Euclidean distance and subsequently comparing it with a threshold or by applying similarity metrics. It is important to note that all regions are hyperrectangles, thus the combined region should be a hyperrectangle as well. In other words, the lower and upper bound for all dimensions should be equal for both regions, except for one dimension where the lower bound in that dimension of one region is equal to the upper bound in the same dimension of the other region. For example, two candidate regions in Fig. 2 are the regions 2 and 3 (but they differ too much in their class distribution to be merged).

Finally, we need to convert our merged decision space back to a decision tree. Unfortunately, the one-to-one mapping from tree to space is not bidirectional, as it is not possible to convert the set of k-dimensional hyperplanes, after the merge operation, to a uniquely defined decision tree. To solve this shortcoming, a heuristic approach is taken which identifies candidate splitting planes to create a node from, and then picks one from these candidates. To select a candidate, a metric (such as information gain) could be used, but this would introduce a bias. Therefore, a candidate is selected randomly. The candidate hyperplanes need to fulfill the constraint that they have no boundaries in all dimensions (or bounds equal to the lower and upper bound of the range of each dimension) except for one. To illustrate this, only one line can be identified as candidate line for the root node in the decision space in Fig. 2. This line is unbounded in the dimension of resting blood pressure but with a value of 147 as maximum heart rate (the line left of region 4).

3.5 Mutation Phase

In each iteration, an individual has a certain probability to be mutated. This can be seen as an 'exploration' parameter to escape local minima. Two mutation operations are defined in GENESIM: either the threshold value of a random node in the decision tree is replaced with another value or two random subtrees are swapped.

3.6 Replacement Phase

The population for the next iteration is created by sorting the individuals by their fitness and only selecting the first *population_size* individuals.

4   Evaluation and Results

The proposed algorithm GENESIM is compared, regarding the predictive performance and model complexity, to two ensemble methods (Random Forests (RF) [12] & eXtreme Gradient Boosting (XGB) [13]) and four decision tree induction algorithms (C4.5 [14], CART [15], GUIDE [16] and QUEST [17]). Moreover, GENESIM is compared to ISM, which we extended with cost-complexity pruning [15]. For this, twelve data sets, having very distinct properties, from the UCI Machine Learning Repository [18] were used. An overview of the characteristics of each data set can be found in Table 1.

When the number of possible combinations was not too high, the hyperparameters of the decision tree induction and ensemble techniques were tuned using a Grid Search technique, else Bayesian optimization was used. Unfortunately, because of a rather high complexity of GENESIM and ISM, hyperparameter optimization could not be applied to these techniques, giving a performance advantage to the other techniques. The ensemble that was transformed

Table 1. Table with the characteristics for each data set. (#cont = number of continuous features, #disc = number of discrete features)

Name	#samples	#cont	#disc	Class distribution
iris	150	4	0	33.3 - 33.3 - 33.3
austra	690	5	9	55.5 - 44.5
cars	1727	0	6	70.0 - 22.2 - 4.0 - 3.8
ecoli	326	5	2	43.6 - 23.6 - 16.0 - 10.7 - 6.1
glass	213	9	0	32.4 - 35.7 - 8.0 - 6.1 - 4.2 - 13.6
heart	269	5	8	55.8 - 44.2
led7	2563	0	7	12.7 - 13.0 - 12.4 - 10.5 - 13.1 - 13.1 - 13.3 - 11.9
lymph	142	0	18	57.0 - 43.0
pima	768	7	1	65.1 - 34.9
vehicle	846	14	4	25.1 - 25.7 - 25.8 - 23.5
wine	177	13	0	32.8 - 40.1 - 27.1
wisconsinBreast	698	0	9	65.5 - 34.5

into a single model by GENESIM was constructed using different induction algorithms (C4.5, CART, QUEST and GUIDE) combined with bagging and boosting. We applied 3-fold cross validation 10 times on each of the data sets and stored the mean accuracy and model complexity for the 3 folds. The mean accuracy and mean model complexity (and their corresponding standard deviations) over these 10 measurements can be found in Tables 2 and 3. In the latter table, the average number of nodes (including the leaves) for the produced decision trees is depicted for each of the decision tree induction algorithms. For the ensemble techniques, the average number of decision trees in the constructed ensemble is depicted. Bootstrap statistical significance testing was applied to construct a Win-Tie-Loss matrix, which can be seen in Fig. 3. Algorithm A wins over B for a certain data set when the mean accuracy is higher than B on that data set and the ρ-value for the bootstrap test is lower than 0.05. When an algorithm has more wins than losses compared to another algorithm, the cell is colored green (and shaded using stripes). Else, the cell is colored red (and shaded using dots). The darker the green, the more wins the algorithm has over the other. Similarly, the darker the red, the more losses an algorithm has over the other.

A few things can be deduced from these matrices and tables. First, we can clearly see that the ensemble techniques RF and XGB have a superior accuracy compared to all other algorithms on these data sets, and that XGB outperforms RF. While the accuracy is indeed better, the increase can be of a rather moderate size (as can be seen in Table 2). However, the resulting model is completely uninterpretable. Second, in terms of accuracy, the proposed GENESIM outperforms all decision tree induction algorithms, except C4.5. Although, GENESIM is very competitive to it. It wins on two data sets while losing on three and has no optimized hyper-parameters, in contrast to C4.5. For each data set, GENESIM used the same hyper-parameters. (such as a limited, fixed amount of iterations and using 50% of the training data as validation data). As can be seen in Fig. 4,

Table 2. Mean accuracies for the different data sets and algorithms using 10 measurements

	XGB	CART	QUEST	GENESIM	RF	ISM	C4.5	GUIDE
heart	0.8257 $\pm$ 0.01σ	0.7441 $\pm$ 0.02σ	0.7585 $\pm$ 0.02σ	0.7982 $\pm$ 0.02σ	0.8129 $\pm$ 0.01σ	0.8024 $\pm$ 0.02σ	0.7877 $\pm$ 0.03σ	0.7829 $\pm$ 0.02σ
led7	0.8018 $\pm$ 0.0σ	0.7997 $\pm$ 0.0σ	0.7986 $\pm$ 0.0σ	0.7926 $\pm$ 0.0σ	0.8027 $\pm$ 0.0σ	0.7996 $\pm$ 0.0σ	0.8012 $\pm$ 0.0σ	0.761 $\pm$ 0.01σ
iris	0.9505 $\pm$ 0.01σ	0.9504 $\pm$ 0.01σ	0.9562 $\pm$ 0.0σ	0.9463 $\pm$ 0.01σ	0.95 $\pm$ 0.01σ	0.9519 $\pm$ 0.01σ	0.9395 $\pm$ 0.01σ	0.9467 $\pm$ 0.01σ
cars	0.9842 $\pm$ 0.0σ	0.9749 $\pm$ 0.0σ	0.9411 $\pm$ 0.01σ	0.9543 $\pm$ 0.01σ	0.9701 $\pm$ 0.01σ	0.9685 $\pm$ 0.0σ	0.966 $\pm$ 0.0σ	0.9426 $\pm$ 0.01σ
ecoli	0.8651 $\pm$ 0.01σ	0.8196 $\pm$ 0.02σ	0.8195 $\pm$ 0.01σ	0.8325 $\pm$ 0.02σ	0.8486 $\pm$ 0.01σ	0.7507 $\pm$ 0.04σ	0.817 $\pm$ 0.03σ	0.8319 $\pm$ 0.01σ
glass	0.7494 $\pm$ 0.02σ	0.6667 $\pm$ 0.03σ	0.649 $\pm$ 0.03σ	0.6696 $\pm$ 0.03σ	0.7526 $\pm$ 0.03σ	0.6489 $\pm$ 0.03σ	0.6763 $\pm$ 0.03σ	0.6557 $\pm$ 0.02σ
austra	0.8686 $\pm$ 0.01σ	0.8506 $\pm$ 0.01σ	0.8547 $\pm$ 0.01σ	0.8553 $\pm$ 0.01σ	0.8663 $\pm$ 0.01σ	0.8557 $\pm$ 0.01σ	0.8528 $\pm$ 0.01σ	0.8582 $\pm$ 0.01σ
vehicle	0.7606 $\pm$ 0.01σ	0.6988 $\pm$ 0.01σ	0.6986 $\pm$ 0.01σ	0.6834 $\pm$ 0.01σ	0.7383 $\pm$ 0.01σ	0.6672 $\pm$ 0.01σ	0.7115 $\pm$ 0.01σ	0.6821 $\pm$ 0.01σ
breast	0.9591 $\pm$ 0.0σ	0.94 $\pm$ 0.01σ	0.947 $\pm$ 0.01σ	0.9496 $\pm$ 0.01σ	0.958 $\pm$ 0.01σ	0.9466 $\pm$ 0.0σ	0.9443 $\pm$ 0.0σ	0.937 $\pm$ 0.01σ
lymph	0.8354 $\pm$ 0.02σ	0.7686 $\pm$ 0.02σ	0.7907 $\pm$ 0.03σ	0.7866 $\pm$ 0.02σ	0.817 $\pm$ 0.02σ	0.7822 $\pm$ 0.03σ	0.7839 $\pm$ 0.03σ	0.7659 $\pm$ 0.04σ
pima	0.7543 $\pm$ 0.01σ	0.7174 $\pm$ 0.02σ	0.7385 $\pm$ 0.01σ	0.7266 $\pm$ 0.01σ	0.7626 $\pm$ 0.01σ	0.7346 $\pm$ 0.01σ	0.7348 $\pm$ 0.01σ	0.7285 $\pm$ 0.02σ
wine	0.9709 $\pm$ 0.01σ	0.9072 $\pm$ 0.01σ	0.9055 $\pm$ 0.03σ	0.9128 $\pm$ 0.03σ	0.9603 $\pm$ 0.01σ	0.8838 $\pm$ 0.01σ	0.9217 $\pm$ 0.01σ	0.8828 $\pm$ 0.03σ

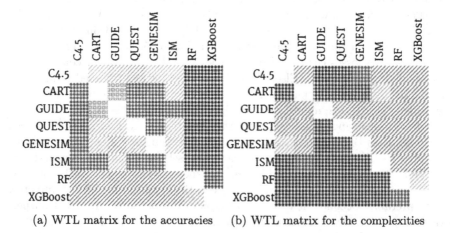

(a) WTL matrix for the accuracies   (b) WTL matrix for the complexities

Fig. 3. Win-Tie-Loss matrices for the different algorithms for accuracies and model complexities (Color figure online)

Table 3. Mean model complexities, expressed as either number of nodes in the resulting decision tree or number of decision trees in the ensemble (*), for the different data sets and algorithms using 10 measurements

	XGB(*)	CART	QUEST	GENESIM	RF(*)	ISM	C4.5	GUIDE
heart	408.4815 ± 188.19σ	35.8148 ± 12.54σ	9.1852 ± 2.97σ	17.4444 ± 4.84σ	448.6113 ± 154.6σ	35.8889 ± 10.71σ	23.5556 ± 6.62σ	9.1481 ± 2.28σ
led7	459.9792 ± 152.17σ	201.9583 ± 1.2σ	57.625 ± 4.91σ	92.0417 ± 17.08σ	516.25 ± 155.4σ	111.2917 ± 15.45σ	58.9583 ± 2.09σ	32.9167 ± 2.55σ
iris	544.5238 ± 144.62σ	12.2857 ± 1.34σ	5.8571 ± 0.59σ	5.9048 ± 0.65σ	453.2381 ± 204.4σ	10.5714 ± 1.91σ	7.3809 ± 1.06σ	5.3333 ± 0.55σ
cars	631.2821 ± 123.71σ	140.1282 ± 2.66σ	45.6667 ± 4.7σ	103.1539 ± 14.42σ	438.4615 ± 178.3σ	131.4102 ± 9.62σ	98.4359 ± 4.6σ	43.6154 ± 5.07σ
ecoli	487.5625 ± 202.89σ	35.6667 ± 11.77σ	14.5833 ± 3.48σ	19.0833 ± 4.27σ	447.0623 ± 147.7σ	60.125 ± 16.06σ	19.25 ± 2.84σ	10.0833 ± 1.43σ
glass	530.7017 ± 179.2σ	57.8421 ± 11.27σ	22.4035 ± 5.66σ	29.6667 ± 5.75σ	486.9825 ± 160σ	80.3684 ± 24.1σ	36.2982 ± 3.09σ	16.1579 ± 2.47σ
austra	433.0392 ± 72.65σ	7.7451 ± 6.19σ	7.902 ± 3.23σ	23.7843 ± 7.37σ	396.3333 ± 181.5σ	38.8824 ± 15.73σ	26.7255 ± 6.82σ	8.2941 ± 3.12σ
vehicle	465.6667 ± 119.44σ	177.1111 ± 22.26σ	81.7778 ± 14.85σ	83.2222 ± 9.68σ	485.2778 ± 146.8σ	345.5556 ± 45.92σ	92.4444 ± 12.43σ	33.2222 ± 8.71σ
breast	563.3333 ± 170.63σ	30.619 ± 7.89σ	12.619 ± 3.73σ	18.5238 ± 3.49σ	395.5714 ± 161.4σ	43.7619 ± 13.31σ	19.4762 ± 2.38σ	10.4286 ± 1.65σ
lymph	608.4375 ± 140.47σ	32.0417 ± 5.75σ	13.5417 ± 3.14σ	14.8333 ± 4.0σ	497.9375 ± 162.3σ	30.9583 ± 6.6σ	16.9583 ± 2.44σ	8.875 ± 2.81σ
pima	180.0556 ± 85.5σ	52.4445 ± 19.8σ	12.0 ± 4.32σ	45.2222 ± 8.53σ	434.8334 ± 68.04σ	101.6667 ± 18.5σ	26.0 ± 5.12σ	8.1111 ± 2.36σ
wine	487.0948 ± 176.94σ	13.4762 ± 1.58σ	9.1905 ± 1.66σ	8.0476 ± 0.93σ	409.2381 ± 116.1σ	33.3809 ± 3.04σ	9.381 ± 0.33σ	6.8095 ± 0.77σ

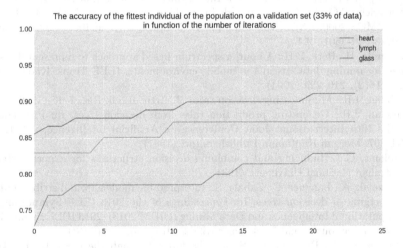

The accuracy of the fittest individual of the population on a validation set (33% of data) in function of the number of iterations

Fig. 4. The fitness (classification rate on a validation set) of the fittest population in function of the number of iterations of GENESIM

running GENESIM for a higher number of iterations could result in a better model. Third, the performance of ISM, which we extended with a post-pruning phase, is rather disappointing. Only GUIDE has a worse classification performance. Moreover, the complexity of the resulting model is higher than the other algorithms as well. Finally, GENESIM produces very interpretable models with a very low model complexity (expressed here as the number of nodes in the tree). The average number of nodes in the resulting tree is lower than in CART and C4.5, but higher than QUEST and GUIDE. But the predictive performance of the two last-mentioned algorithms is much lower than GENESIM.

5 Conclusion

In this paper, GENESIM is proposed, a genetic approach for exploiting the positive properties of ensembles while keeping the result a single, interpretable model. GENESIM is ideally suited to support the decision-making process of experts in critical domains. Results show that in most cases, an increased predictive performance compared to naive induction algorithms can be achieved, while keeping a very similar model complexity. Results of GENESIM can still be improved by reducing the computational complexity of our algorithm, allowing hyperparameter optimization and enabling our technique to run for more iterations in a feasible amount of time.

References

1. Slonim, D.K.: From patterns to pathways. Nat. Genetics **32**, 502–508 (2002)
2. Dietterich, T.G.: Ensemble methods in machine learning. In: Kittler, J., Roli, F. (eds.) MCS 2000. LNCS, vol. 1857, pp. 1–15. Springer, Heidelberg (2000). doi:10. 1007/3-540-45014-9_1
3. Kargupta, H., Park, B.H.: A Fourier spectrum-based approach to represent decision trees for mining data streams in mobile environments. IEEE Trans. Knowl. Data Eng. **16**(2), 216–229 (2004)
4. Quinlan, J.R.: Miniboosting decision trees. J. Artif. Intell. Res. 1–15 (1998)
5. Quinlan, J.R.: Generating production rules from decision trees. In: Proceedings of the 10th International Joint Conference on Artificial Intelligence, vol. 1, pp. 304–307. Morgan Kaufmann Publishers Inc. (1987)
6. Williams, G.J.: Inducing and combining decision structures for expert systems. Australian National University (1991)
7. Andrzejak, A., Langner, F., Zabala, S.: Interpretable models from distributed data via merging of decision trees. In: Proceedings of the 2013 IEEE Symposium on Computational Intelligence and Data Mining (CIDM 2013)–2013 IEEE Symposium Series on Computational Intelligence (SSCI 2013), pp. 1–9 (2013)
8. Van Assche, A., Blockeel, H.: Seeing the forest through the trees. In: Blockeel, H., Ramon, J., Shavlik, J., Tadepalli, P. (eds.) ILP 2007. LNCS, vol. 4894, pp. 269–279. Springer, Heidelberg (2008). doi:10.1007/978-3-540-78469-2_26
9. Deng, H.: Interpreting tree ensembles with intrees. arXiv preprint arXiv:1408.5456 (2014)
10. Holland, J.H.: Adaptation in Natural and Artificial Systems. University of Michigan Press, Ann Arbor (1975)
11. Barros, R.C., Basgalupp, M.P., De Carvalho, A.C., Freitas, A.A.: A survey of evolutionary algorithms for decision-tree induction. IEEE Trans. Syst. Man Cybern. Part C Appl. Rev. **42**(3), 291–312 (2012)

12. Breiman, L.: Random forests. Mach. Learn. **45**(5), 1–35 (1999)
13. Chen, T., Guestrin, C.: Xgboost: a scalable tree boosting system. arXiv preprint arXiv:1603.02754 (2016)
14. Quinlan, J.R.: C4.5: Programs for Machine Learning. Morgan Kaufmann Publishers Inc., San Francisco (1993)
15. Breiman, L., Friedman, J., Stone, C.J., Olshen, R.A.: Classification and Regression Trees. Chapman and Hall/CRC, Boca Raton (1984)
16. Loh, W.-Y.: Improving the precision of classification trees. Ann. Appl. Stat. 1710–1737 (2009)
17. Loh, W.-Y., Shih, Y.-S.: Split selection methods for classification trees. Stat. Sinica **7**(4), 815–840 (1997)
18. Lichman, M.: UCI machine learning repository (2013)

Self-adaptive Weighted Extreme Learning Machine for Imbalanced Classification Problems

Hao Long, Yulin He$^{(\boxtimes)}$, Joshua Zhexue Huang, and Qiang Wang

Big Data Institute, College of Computer Science and Software Engineering,
Shenzhen University, Shenzhen 518060, China
`longhao1@email.szu.edu.cn, csylhe@126.com,`
`{zx.huang,wangqiang}@szu.edu.cn`

Abstract. A self-adaptive weighted extreme learning machine (SawELM) is proposed in this paper to deal with the imbalanced binary-class classification problems. SawELM calculates the output-layer weights based on a newly-designed self-adaptive mechanism which includes the following two modules: one is to gradually reduce the weights of wrongly-classified training instances and the other is to dynamically update the outputs of these wrongly-classified instances. On 50 imbalanced binary-class data sets selected from KEEL repository, we compare the accuracy, G-mean, and F-measure of SawELM with unweighted ELM (UnWELM) and weighted ELM (WELM). The experimental results show that the newly-designed self-adaptive mechanism is effective and SawELM obviously improves the imbalanced classification performance of WELM. SawWLM obtains the significantly higher G-mean and F-measure than UnWELM and WELM. Meanwhile, the accuracy of SawELM is better than WELM and comparable to UnWELM.

Keywords: Imbalanced classification · Weighted extreme learning machine · Unweighted extreme learning machine · G-mean · F-measure

1 Introduction

The imbalanced classification is an important and attractive research topic in the field of machine learning, because the unequal distribution between data set classes is a very common phenomenon in the real world and can significantly compromise the performance of most standard classification algorithms [7]. The imbalanced data sets can be easily found in many practical applications, e.g., click-through rate prediction of search engine, commodity recommendation in the area of e-commerce, credit card fraud detection, and network attack detection, etc. The standard classification algorithms assume that the class distribution is balanced and thus most of them make the unfavorable prediction for minority class. In reality, the cost of misclassifying the minority class instances as the majority class instances is always higher than the cost of contrary case [20]. For example, it is very dangerous to diagnose the "cancerous" patients (minority class) as "noncancerous" persons (majority class). Therefore, we require a

© Springer International Publishing AG 2017
U Kang et al. (Eds.): PAKDD 2017 Workshops, LNAI 10526, pp. 116–128, 2017.
DOI: 10.1007/978-3-319-67274-8_11

learning method which will train a classifier having the high predictive accuracy for minority class without severely degrading the predictive accuracy of majority class.

Two representative learning methods focusing on imbalanced classification are the sampling and cost-sensitive learning. The sampling methods firstly balance the imbalanced data set by removing the majority instances (random under-sampling) [13] or adding the minority instances (random over-sampling) [6] and then train a classifier based on the balanced data set. The problems of sampling methods are that the under-sampling easily results in the over-fitting of classifier and the over-sampling may cause the classifier to miss the important information of majority class [7]. The objective of cost-sensitive methods is to train a classifier that minimizes the overall "classification cost" on the imbalanced training data set [14]. A cost matrix should be defined in the cost-sensitive method to represent the cost of classifying instances from one class to another. Usually, the cost of misclassifying the minority class instances is higher than the cost of misclassifying the majority class instances. The representative cost-sensitive learning paradigms include the cost-sensitive ensemble learning [18], cost-sensitive neural network [20], and cost-sensitive decision tree [19], etc. Though we only briefly introduce two typical strategies to deal with the imbalanced classification, many other techniques also exist for solving this problem, e.g., ensemble learning-based [5,11] and active learning-based [3,4] imbalanced classification methods. More detailed concepts and algorithms on imbalanced classification can be found from the literatures [7,8].

Recently, the extreme learning machine (ELM)-based imbalanced classification methods have drawn a lot of attention from academia and industry due to the fast training speed and good predictive performance of ELM. ELM [9,10] is a special single hidden-layer feed-forward neural networks of which the input-layer weights are randomly selected from a given interval (e.g., $[0,1]$) and the output-layer weights are analytically calculated by calculating *Moore-Penrose* generalized inverse of hidden-layer output matrix. Due to avoiding the iterative training of weights and complex tuning of learning parameters, ELM has the extremely fast training speed and obtains the good predictive performances in many fields [12,16,17,21] including the imbalanced classification discussed in this study. In 2013, Zong et al. [21] gave the first ELM-based imbalance classification model named weighted ELM (WELM), where a diagonal weight matrix associated with each training instance was introduced into the constrained optimization problem of unweighted ELM (UnWELM) [9]. The objective of weighting instances is to "*strengthen the impact of minority class while weaken the impact of majority class.* [21]" on the classification performance of trained ELM model. In 2014, Li et al. [12] proposed a boosting weighted ELM which tried to improve the weighting scheme of WELM by embedding it into an modified AdaBoost framework. Yang et al. in 2015 [16] designed an imbalanced ELM algorithm for imbalanced binary-class classification problem by modifying the probability density functions of predictive outputs and retraining the classifier with the modified training data set. Xiao et al. in 2016 [15] also presented an imbalanced ELM algorithm which employed two different regularization terms in the constrained optimization problem of unweighted ELM (UnWELM) [9]. These two regularization terms were associated with the predictive errors of majority and minority classes, respectively. The ELM-based imbalance classification models mentioned above demonstrate the feasibility of using ELM to deal with the imbalanced classification problems.

In this paper, we focus on improving the classical WELM [21] by analyzing the impact of weight factors on the predictive performance of WELM. Motivated by further improving the predictive performance of WELM, a self-adaptive weighted extreme learning machine (SawELM) algorithm is proposed to deal with the imbalanced binary-class classification problems. SawELM is a single hidden-layer feed-forward neural network of which the input-layer weights are randomly selected from interval $[0, 1]$ and the output-layer weights are determined based on a newly-designed self-adaptive mechanism. The self-adaptive mechanism of SawELM mainly includes two parts: one is to gradually reduce the weights of wrongly-classified training instances and the other is to dynamically adjust the real outputs of these wrongly-classified instances. We compare the accuracy, G-mean, and F-measure of SawELM with UnWELM and WELM on 50 imbalanced binary-class data sets selected from KEEL repository [1,2]. The experimental results show that SawELM obviously improves the imbalanced classification performance of WELM. SawELM obtains the significantly higher G-mean and F-measure than UnWELM and WELM. In addition, the accuracy of SawELM is better than WELM and comparable to UnWELM.

The remainder of this paper is organized as follows. In Sect. 2, we briefly introduce the weighted extreme learning machine (WELM). The self-adaptive weighted extreme learning machine (SawELM) is presented in Sect. 3. In Sect. 4, we report the experimental comparisons that demonstrate the feasibility and effectiveness of SawELM. Finally, we give our conclusions and suggestions for further research in Sect. 5.

2   Weighted Extreme Learning Machine (WELM)

For an ELM algorithm, the main task is to determine its output-layer weights. Before the basic concepts of WELM [21] are introduced, we firstly describe the unweighted ELM (UnWELM) [9]. For an given imbalanced binary-class data set

$$D = \left\{ (\bar{x}_n, \bar{y}_n) \middle| \begin{array}{l} \bar{x}_n = (x_{n1}, x_{n2}, \cdots, x_{nD}), \\ \bar{y}_n = (y_{n1}, y_{n2}) = \begin{cases} (1,0), \text{ if } \bar{x}_n \text{ belongs to the majority class} \\ (0,1), \text{ if } \bar{x}_n \text{ belongs to the minority class} \end{cases} \end{array} \right\},$$

where, $n = 1, 2, \cdots, N$, N is the number of instances, D is the number of attributes, and the numbers of instances belonging to the majority and minority classes are N_{Maj} and N_{Min} ($N_{Maj} + N_{Min} = N$), respectively. UnWELM [9] randomly selects the input-layer weights and hidden-layer biases from $[0, 1]$ and analytically determines the output-layer weights as

$$\beta_{\text{UnWELM}} = \begin{cases} H^T \left(\frac{I}{C} + HH^T \right)^{-1} Y, \text{ if } N < L \\ \left(\frac{I}{C} + H^T H \right)^{-1} H^T Y, \text{ if } N \geq L \end{cases} \tag{1}$$

by solving the following constrained optimization problem

$$\text{Minimize} : L_{\text{UnWELM}} = \frac{1}{2}\|\beta\|^2 + \frac{C}{2}\sum_{n=1}^{N}\left\|\bar{\xi}_n\right\|^2 ,$$
$$\text{Subject to} : \bar{\xi}_n = \bar{y}_n - \text{h}(\bar{x}_n)\beta, \ n = 1, 2, \cdots, N \quad (2)$$

where,

$$\text{H} = \begin{bmatrix} \text{h}(\bar{x}_1) \\ \text{h}(\bar{x}_2) \\ \vdots \\ \text{h}(\bar{x}_N) \end{bmatrix} = \begin{bmatrix} h_1(\bar{x}_1) & h_2(\bar{x}_1) & \cdots & h_L(\bar{x}_1) \\ h_1(\bar{x}_2) & h_2(\bar{x}_2) & \cdots & h_L(\bar{x}_2) \\ \vdots & \vdots & \ddots & \vdots \\ h_1(\bar{x}_N) & h_2(\bar{x}_N) & \cdots & h_L(\bar{x}_N) \end{bmatrix}$$

is the hidden-layer output matrix, $h_l(\bar{x}_n) = g(\bar{\alpha}_l \bar{x}_n + b_l)$ is the output of the l-th $(l = 1, 2, \cdots, L)$ hidden-layer node corresponding to the n-th training instance $\bar{x}_n$, $g(v) = \frac{1}{1+\exp(-v)}, v \in (-\infty, +\infty)$ is the sigmoid activation function,

$$\alpha = \begin{bmatrix} \bar{\alpha}_1 \ \bar{\alpha}_2 \cdots \bar{\alpha}_L \end{bmatrix} = \begin{bmatrix} \alpha_{11} & \alpha_{21} & \cdots & \alpha_{L1} \\ \alpha_{12} & \alpha_{22} & \cdots & \alpha_{L2} \\ \vdots & \vdots & \ddots & \vdots \\ \alpha_{1D} & \alpha_{2D} & \cdots & \alpha_{LD} \end{bmatrix}$$

are the input-layer weights, $\bar{b} = \begin{bmatrix} b_1 \ b_2 \cdots b_L \end{bmatrix}^{\text{T}}$ are the hidden-layer biases, L is the number of hidden-layer nodes, and $C > 0$ is the regularization factor.

UnWELM doesn't consider the class distribution of imbalanced data set when determining the output-layer weights β. In order to improve the predictive capability of UnWELM on the minority class instances, Zong et al. proposed a weighted ELM (WELM) algorithm [21] by modifying the constrained optimization problem Eq. (2) of UnWELM as

$$\text{Minimize} : L_{\text{UnWELM}} = \frac{1}{2}\|\beta\|^2 + \frac{C}{2}\sum_{n=1}^{N} w_{nn}\left\|\bar{\xi}_n\right\|^2 ,$$
$$\text{Subject to} : \bar{\xi}_n = \bar{y}_n - \text{h}(\bar{x}_n)\beta, \ n = 1, 2, \cdots, N \quad (3)$$

where,

$$w_{nn} = \begin{cases} \frac{1}{N_{Maj}}, & \text{if } \bar{x}_n \text{ belongs to the majority class} \\ \frac{1}{N_{Min}}, & \text{if } \bar{x}_n \text{ belongs to the minority class} \end{cases} \quad (4)$$

is the weight factor corresponding to the n-th training instance $\bar{x}_n$. By solving the optimization problem Eq. (3), the output-layer weights of WELM are calculated as

$$\beta_{\text{WELM}} = \begin{cases} \text{H}^{\text{T}}(\frac{\text{I}}{C} + \text{WHH}^{\text{T}})^{-1}\text{WY}, & \text{if } N < L \\ (\frac{\text{I}}{C} + \text{H}^{\text{T}}\text{WH})^{-1}\text{H}^{\text{T}}\text{WY}, & \text{if } N \geq L \end{cases}, \quad (5)$$

where, $\text{W} = \text{diag}(w_{11}, w_{22}, \cdots, w_{NN})$ is a $N \times N$ diagonal weight matrix. The experimental results [21] demonstrate that WELM indeed obtains the better predictive performance on the minority class instances than UnWELM by weakening the impact of majority class instances and meanwhile strengthening the impact of minority class instances.

3   Self-adaptive Weighted Extreme Learning Machine (SawELM)

Before our imbalanced classification model is provided, we briefly analyze the main reason why WELM improve the predictive performance of UnWELM. For β_{WELM} as shown in Eq. (5), we further extend it and then derive the following formula as

$$\beta_{\text{WELM}} = \left(\frac{I}{C} + H^T W H\right)^{-1} H^T W Y = \left(\frac{I}{C} + H^T \sqrt{W}\sqrt{W}H\right)^{-1} H^T \sqrt{W}\sqrt{W}Y$$

$$= \left[\frac{I}{C} + \left(\sqrt{W}H\right)^T \left(\sqrt{W}H\right)\right]^{-1} \left(\sqrt{W}H\right)^T \left(\sqrt{W}Y\right)$$

(6)

for $N \geq L$, where $\sqrt{W} = \text{diag}\left(\sqrt{w_{11}}, \sqrt{w_{22}}, \cdots, \sqrt{w_{NN}}\right)$. By comparing β_{WELM} in Eq. (6) with β_{UnWELM} in Eq. (1), we can find that the main difference between WELM and UnWELM is that WELM uses the weight matrix $\sqrt{W}$ to weight the hidden-layer output matrix H and the data output matrix Y, i.e.,

$$\sqrt{W}H = \begin{bmatrix} \sqrt{w_{11}}h_1(\bar{x}_1) & \sqrt{w_{11}}h_2(\bar{x}_1) & \cdots & \sqrt{w_{11}}h_L(\bar{x}_1) \\ \sqrt{w_{22}}h_1(\bar{x}_2) & \sqrt{w_{22}}h_2(\bar{x}_2) & \cdots & \sqrt{w_{22}}h_L(\bar{x}_2) \\ \vdots & \vdots & \ddots & \vdots \\ \sqrt{w_{NN}}h_1(\bar{x}_N) & \sqrt{w_{NN}}h_2(\bar{x}_N) & \cdots & \sqrt{w_{NN}}h_L(\bar{x}_N) \end{bmatrix}$$

(7)

and

$$\sqrt{W}Y = \begin{bmatrix} \sqrt{w_{11}}y_{11} & \sqrt{w_{11}}y_{12} \\ \sqrt{w_{22}}y_{21} & \sqrt{w_{22}}y_{22} \\ \vdots & \vdots \\ \sqrt{w_{NN}}y_{N1} & \sqrt{w_{NN}}y_{N2} \end{bmatrix}.$$

(8)

By weighting the hidden-layer output matrix H and the data output matrix Y, WELM moves the classification boundary towards the majority class [21] and thus increases the probability of correctly classifying the minority class instances. WELM improves the predictive performance of UnWELM on the imbalanced data set by assigning the smaller weights for majority class instances and the larger weights for minority class instances. However, there is still room to improve the imbalanced classification capability of WELM. The instances belonging to the same class are treated equally in WELM, i.e., the same weights are assigned to the different instances in the same class. This weighting scheme can't effectively deal with the imbalanced class distribution as shown in Fig. 1(a). Although WELM makes the classification boundary move towards the majority class, WELM can't correctly classify the minority class instance $\bar{x}_{\min}$ (Fig. 1(b)). This section gives an improved version of WELM to further enhance the imbalanced classification capability of WELM. The improved WELM as summarized in Algorithm 1 is called the self-adaptive weighted extreme learning machine (SawELM).

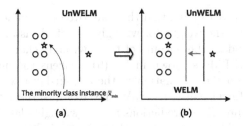

Fig. 1. The classification boundaries of UnWELM and WELM. For simplicity we use the straight lines to represent the classification boundaries which may be curves for the true data sets.

Algorithm 1. SawWLM

1: **Input:** The imbalanced binary-class data set $D^{(0)}$; the random input-layer weights α and hidden-layer biases $\bar{b}$ selected from $[0, 1]$; the number L of hidden-layer nodes; the regularization factor C.

2: **Output:** The output-layer weights β_{SawELM} of SawELM.

3: Use the original training data set $D^{(0)}$ and weight matrix $W^{(0)}$ as shown in Eq. (4) to train the initial WELM model WELM$^{(0)}$;

4: Calculate the output-layer weight matrix $\beta_{WELM}^{(0)}$ according to Eq. (5);

5: Use the training data set $D^{(0)}$ to evaluate the G-mean value $G^{(0)}$ of WELM$^{(0)}$;

6: $k = 0$;

7: **repeat**

8:     Find the instances $\bar{x}_1^{(k)}, \bar{x}_2^{(k)}, \cdots, \bar{x}_{N^{(k)}}^{(k)}$ which are wrongly classified by WELM$^{(k)}$;

9:     **for** $i = 1$ to $N^{(k)}$ **do**

10:        Adjust the weight of wrongly-classified instance $\bar{x}_i^{(k)}$:

$$w\left(\bar{x}_i^{(k)}\right) = \begin{cases} \frac{1}{N_{Maj}+(k+1)}, & \text{if } \bar{x}_i^{(k)} \text{ belongs to the majority class} \\ \frac{1}{N_{Min}+(k+1)}, & \text{if } \bar{x}_i^{(k)} \text{ belongs to the minority class} \end{cases} ; \quad (9)$$

11:        Update the output of wrongly-classified instance $\bar{x}_i^{(k)}$:

$$\bar{y}_i^{(k)} = \begin{cases} (1+(k+1),0), & \text{if } \bar{x}_i^{(k)} \text{ belongs to the majority class} \\ (0,1+(k+1)), & \text{if } \bar{x}_i^{(k)} \text{ belongs to the minority class} \end{cases} ; \quad (10)$$

12:     **end for**

13:     $k = k + 1$;

14:     Use the updated training data set $D^{(k)}$ and the adjusted weight matrix $W^{(k)}$ to train the WELM model WELM$^{(k)}$;

15:     Calculate the output-layer weight matrix $\beta_{WELM}^{(k)}$ according to Eq. (5);

16:     Use the training data set $D^{(k)}$ to evaluate the G-mean value $G^{(k)}$ of WELM$^{(k)}$;

17: **until** $\left\{ G^{(k)} < G^{(k-1)} \right\}$

18: WELM$^{(k-1)}$ with the output-layer weight matrix $\beta_{WELM}^{(k-1)}$ is the trained SawELM of which the output-layer weights $\beta_{SawELM} = \beta_{WELM}^{(k-1)}$.

From Algorithm 1 we can find that there are two key modules in SawELM: one is to gradually adjust the weights of wrongly-classified instances and the other is to dynamically update the outputs of these wrongly-classified instances. The first module of SawELM as shown in Eq. (9) weakens the impact of wrongly-classified instances on the calculation of the output-layer weights. The second module as shown in Eq. (10) instructs SaWELM to adjust the output-layer weights in order that the appropriate predictions for the wrongly-classified instances can be obtained. We provide an example to show the feasibility of SawELM, i.e., the predictive output of WELM can be changed when WELM is improved according to Algorithm 1. Assume that there is an imbalanced data set which includes 2 minority class instances and 6 majority class instances. Let $C = 2^{10}$ and $L = 10$ for WELM and SawELM which have the same hidden-layer output matrix, i.e.,

$$H = \begin{bmatrix} h_1 \\ h_2 \\ h_3 \\ h_4 \\ h_5 \\ h_6 \\ h_7 \\ h_8 \end{bmatrix} = \begin{bmatrix} 0.0174 & 0.0170 & 0.0158 & 0.0158 & 0.0169 & 0.0165 & 0.0168 & 0.0160 & 0.0178 & 0.0178 \\ 0.0168 & 0.0173 & 0.0157 & 0.0172 & 0.0163 & 0.0173 & 0.0155 & 0.0175 & 0.0150 & 0.0164 \\ 0.0180 & 0.0186 & 0.0182 & 0.0170 & 0.0182 & 0.0185 & 0.0195 & 0.0182 & 0.0181 & 0.0176 \\ 0.0197 & 0.0196 & 0.0180 & 0.0190 & 0.0187 & 0.0182 & 0.0183 & 0.0183 & 0.0185 & 0.0173 \\ 0.0179 & 0.0189 & 0.0191 & 0.0193 & 0.0187 & 0.0195 & 0.0199 & 0.0193 & 0.0198 & 0.0193 \\ 0.0193 & 0.0194 & 0.0171 & 0.0170 & 0.0190 & 0.0173 & 0.0194 & 0.0174 & 0.0171 & 0.0197 \\ 0.0197 & 0.0191 & 0.0190 & 0.0179 & 0.0190 & 0.0171 & 0.0190 & 0.0191 & 0.0195 & 0.0177 \\ 0.0198 & 0.0191 & 0.0196 & 0.0181 & 0.0196 & 0.0199 & 0.0190 & 0.0171 & 0.0188 & 0.0190 \end{bmatrix}.$$

The data output matrices of WELM and SawELM after five-times iterations are

$$Y_{WELM} = \begin{bmatrix} 0 & 1 \\ 0 & 1 \\ 1 & 0 \\ 1 & 0 \\ 1 & 0 \\ 1 & 0 \\ 1 & 0 \\ 1 & 0 \end{bmatrix} \text{ and } Y_{SawELM} = \begin{bmatrix} 0 & 1+5 \\ 0 & 1 \\ 1 & 0 \\ 1 & 0 \\ 1 & 0 \\ 1 & 0 \\ 1 & 0 \\ 1 & 0 \end{bmatrix}.$$

The weight matrices of WELM and SawELM are

$$W_{WELM} = \text{diag}\left(\frac{1}{2}, \frac{1}{2}, \frac{1}{6}, \frac{1}{6}, \frac{1}{6}, \frac{1}{6}, \frac{1}{6}, \frac{1}{6}\right) \text{ and } W_{SawELM} = \text{diag}\left(\frac{1}{2+5}, \frac{1}{2}, \frac{1}{6}, \frac{1}{6}, \frac{1}{6}, \frac{1}{6}, \frac{1}{6}, \frac{1}{6}\right).$$

Then, the predictive outputs of the first minority class instance can be calculated as

$$y_{WELM} = (0.4331, 0.3867) \text{ and } y_{SawELM} = (0.5038, 0.6133).$$

We can see that SawELM $(0.5038 < 0.6133)$ predicts the correct class for the first minority class instance which is wrongly classified by WELM $(0.4331 > 0.3867)$.

4   Experimental Validation

In this section we select 50 KEEL [1,2] imbalanced binary-class data sets as shown in Table 1 to demonstrate the feasibility and effectiveness of SawELM. In Table 1 IR means the imbalanced ratio (IR) of data set, i.e., $\text{IR} = \frac{N_{Maj}}{N_{Min}}$. We compare the testing G-mean, testing F-measure, testing accuracy, and training time of SawELM with UnWELM [9] and WELM [21]. Each data set is randomly

Table 1. 50 KEEL [1,2] imbalanced binary-class data sets

No	Data set	Attributes (D)	Instances (N)	Majority class (N_{Maj})	Minority class (N_{Min})	IR ($\frac{N_{Maj}}{N_{Min}}$)
1	Ecoli-0-1-3-7-vs-2-6	7	281	274	7	39.14
2	Ecoli-0-1-4-6-vs-5	6	280	260	20	13
3	Ecoli-0-1-4-7-vs-2-3-5-6	7	336	307	29	10.59
4	Ecoli-0-1-4-7-vs-5-6	6	332	307	25	12.28
5	Ecoli-0-2-3-4-vs-5	7	202	182	20	9.1
6	Ecoli-0-2-6-7-vs-3-5	7	224	202	22	9.18
7	Ecoli-0-3-4-6-vs-5	7	205	185	20	9.25
8	Ecoli-0-3-4-7-vs-5-6	7	257	232	25	9.28
9	Ecoli-0-3-4-vs-5	7	200	180	20	9
10	Ecoli-0-4-6-vs-5	6	203	183	20	9.15
11	Ecoli-0-6-7-vs-5	6	220	200	20	10
12	Ecoli3	7	336	301	35	8.6
13	Glass-0-1-2-3-vs-4-5-6	9	214	163	51	3.2
14	Glass-0-1-4-6-vs-2	9	205	188	17	11.06
15	Glass-0-1-5-vs-2	9	172	155	17	9.12
16	Glass-0-1-6-vs-2	9	192	175	17	10.29
17	Glass0	9	214	144	70	2.06
18	Glass1	9	214	138	76	1.82
19	Glass2	9	214	197	17	11.59
20	Glass4	9	214	201	13	15.46
21	Glass5	9	214	205	9	22.78
22	Glass6	9	214	185	29	6.38
23	New-thyroid1	5	215	180	35	5.14
24	Page-blocks-1-3-vs-4	10	472	444	28	15.86
25	Page-blocks0	10	5472	4913	559	8.79
26	Pima	8	768	500	268	1.87
27	Poker-8-vs-6	10	1477	1460	17	85.88
28	Segment0	19	2308	1979	329	6.02
29	Shuttle-2-vs-5	9	3316	3267	49	66.67
30	Vehicle0	18	846	647	199	3.25
31	Vehicle1	18	846	629	217	2.9
32	Vehicle3	18	846	634	212	2.99
33	Winequality-red-3-vs-5	11	691	681	10	68.1
34	Winequality-red-4	11	1599	1546	53	29.17
35	Winequality-red-8-vs-6-7	11	855	837	18	46.5
36	Winequality-red-8-vs-6	11	656	638	18	35.44
37	Winequality-white-3-9-vs-5	11	1482	1457	25	58.28
38	Winequality-white-3-vs-7	11	900	880	20	44
39	Yeast-0-2-5-6-vs-3-7-8-9	8	1004	905	99	9.14
40	Yeast-0-2-5-7-9-vs-3-6-8	8	1004	905	99	9.14
41	Yeast-0-3-5-9-vs-7-8	8	506	456	50	9.12
42	Yeast-0-5-6-7-9-vs-4	8	528	477	51	9.35
43	Yeast-1-2-8-9-vs-7	8	947	917	30	30.57
44	Yeast-1-4-5-8-vs-7	8	693	663	30	22.1
45	Yeast-1-vs-7	7	459	429	30	14.3
46	Yeast-2-vs-4	8	514	463	51	9.08
47	Yeast-2-vs-8	8	482	462	20	23.1
48	Yeast4	8	1484	1433	51	28.1
49	Yeast5	8	1484	1440	44	32.73
50	Yeast6	8	1484	1449	35	41.4

divided into two parts: 70% of instances are used as training data and the other 30% are testing data. The whole data, training data, and testing data have the approximately equal class distribution. We use the training data to train the different ELM models and use the testing data to test their G-means, F-measures, and accuracies. This procedure is repeated 10 times and the means of 10-times runs are used as the final experimental results.

G-mean, F-measure, and accuracy are three commonly-used evaluation metrics to check the predictive performance of an imbalanced classification algorithm $\mathbb{A}$. Assume that there are N instances in the testing data set which includes N_{Maj} majority class instances and N_{Min} minority class instances. For the algorithm $\mathbb{A}$, the numbers of correctly-classified majority class instances, correctly-classified minority class instances, wrongly-classified majority class instances, and wrongly-classified minority class instances are TP, TN, FN, and FP, respectively. Then, G-mean, F-measure, and accuracy of $\mathbb{A}$ are calculated as

$$\text{G-mean} = \sqrt{\frac{TP}{TP+FN} \times \frac{TN}{TN+FP}}; \tag{11}$$

$$\text{F-measure} = \frac{2TP}{2TP+FN+FP}; \tag{12}$$

and

$$\text{Accuracy} = \frac{TP+TN}{N}. \tag{13}$$

We select 2 different parameter pairs $(C, L) = \left(2^{20}, 200\right)$ and $(C, L) = \left(2^{20}, 500\right)$ to compare the testing G-mean, testing F-measure, testing accuracy, and training time of SawELM with UnWELM [9] and WELM [21]. The comparative results are summarized in Tables 2 and 3. From these tables we can clearly find that (1) the testing G-means and F-measures of SawELM are better than UnWELM and WELM and (2) the testing accuracy of SawELM is better than WELM. For example, when $(C, L) = \left(2^{20}, 200\right)$, the testing G-means of SawELM on Ecoli-0-3-4-7-vs-5-6 and Glass-0-1-4-6-vs-2 data sets are 0.989 and 0.945, while the testing G-means of WELM on these two data sets are 0.931 and 0.914 which are obviously smaller than SawELM; when $(C, L) = \left(2^{20}, 500\right)$, the testing F-measures of SawELM on Ecoli-0-6-7-vs-5 and Yeast-1-2-8-9-vs-7 data sets are 0.986 and 0.865, while the testing F-measures of WELM on these two data sets are 0.926 and 0.807. The main reason that SawELM obtains the higher testing G-mean and testing F-measure is that SawELM increases the number of minority class instances which are correctly classified or reduces the number of minority class instances which are wrongly classified. Assume that G-mean$_{\text{WELM}}$ and G-mean$_{\text{SawELM}}$ are the testing G-means of WELM and SawELM on a given data set, where

$$\text{G-mean}_{\text{WELM}} = \sqrt{\frac{TP}{TP+FN} \times \frac{TN_{\text{WELM}}}{TN_{\text{WELM}}+FP_{\text{WELM}}}}$$

and

$$\text{G-mean}_{\text{SawELM}} = \sqrt{\frac{TP}{TP+FN} \times \frac{TN_{\text{SawELM}}}{TN_{\text{SawELM}}+FP_{\text{SawELM}}}}.$$

Table 2. The comparative results among UnWELM, WELM, and SawELM with $(C, L) = (2^{20}, 200)$

Data set	Testing G-mean			Testing F-measure			Testing accuracy			Training time			Iterations
	UnWELM	WELM	SawELM	UnWELM	WELM	SawELM	UnWELM	WELM	SawELM	UnWELM	WELM	SawELM	
1	0.812±0.317	0.964±0.012	0.969±0.012	0.800±0.322	0.963±0.013	0.968±0.013	0.994±0.008	0.931±0.023	0.940±0.023	0.005±0.001	0.006±0.000	0.049±0.004	8.000±1.000
2	0.910±0.075	0.986±0.006	0.993±0.006	0.904±0.082	0.986±0.006	0.993±0.006	0.988±0.010	0.975±0.010	0.987±0.010	0.005±0.001	0.006±0.001	0.048±0.004	7.000±0.000
3	0.884±0.081	0.920±0.047	0.919±0.045	0.875±0.090	0.918±0.049	0.917±0.047	0.983±0.012	0.961±0.012	0.959±0.014	0.005±0.000	0.008±0.001	0.055±0.005	7.000±0.000
4	0.868±0.056	0.979±0.032	0.987±0.005	0.859±0.064	0.979±0.033	0.987±0.005	0.983±0.007	0.987±0.008	0.976±0.010	0.005±0.000	0.007±0.000	0.058±0.006	7.000±0.000
5	0.956±0.046	0.982±0.010	0.989±0.007	0.955±0.048	0.982±0.011	0.989±0.008	0.992±0.009	0.968±0.018	0.980±0.013	0.004±0.001	0.004±0.000	0.033±0.001	7.000±0.000
6	0.873±0.065	0.930±0.063	0.988±0.008	0.864±0.072	0.927±0.067	0.988±0.008	0.979±0.011	0.973±0.020	0.979±0.015	0.004±0.001	0.005±0.001	0.040±0.003	8.000±1.000
7	0.945±0.064	0.990±0.007	0.991±0.006	0.942±0.068	0.990±0.007	0.991±0.006	0.987±0.015	0.982±0.012	0.984±0.011	0.003±0.000	0.005±0.001	0.031±0.002	7.000±1.000
8	0.888±0.114	0.931±0.068	0.989±0.007	0.876±0.131	0.927±0.073	0.989±0.007	0.982±0.018	0.975±0.018	0.980±0.013	0.004±0.001	0.006±0.001	0.046±0.003	8.000±0.000
9	0.938±0.061	0.992±0.007	0.993±0.007	0.935±0.065	0.992±0.007	0.992±0.007	0.988±0.011	0.985±0.012	0.987±0.013	0.004±0.000	0.004±0.000	0.031±0.002	7.000±1.000
10	0.965±0.045	0.989±0.007	0.993±0.006	0.964±0.047	0.989±0.007	0.993±0.006	0.993±0.009	0.980±0.013	0.987±0.011	0.004±0.000	0.005±0.001	0.031±0.002	7.000±0.000
11	0.938±0.061	0.945±0.044	0.985±0.011	0.935±0.065	0.944±0.046	0.985±0.011	0.989±0.010	0.971±0.015	0.973±0.020	0.004±0.000	0.007±0.001	0.042±0.003	8.000±1.000
12	0.790±0.052	0.915±0.029	0.928±0.027	0.771±0.061	0.913±0.028	0.927±0.027	0.945±0.012	0.888±0.023	0.911±0.022	0.005±0.000	0.007±0.001	0.065±0.011	8.000±1.000
13	0.990±0.014	0.960±0.017	0.980±0.009	0.990±0.014	0.960±0.017	0.980±0.010	0.992±0.008	0.954±0.014	0.970±0.014	0.004±0.000	0.005±0.001	0.035±0.001	7.000±0.000
14	0.222±0.234	0.914±0.038	0.945±0.022	0.166±0.175	0.911±0.039	0.943±0.023	0.918±0.011	0.864±0.040	0.902±0.038	0.004±0.001	0.005±0.000	0.039±0.001	8.000±0.000
15	0.589±0.183	0.924±0.022	0.945±0.017	0.512±0.225	0.921±0.023	0.943±0.018	0.935±0.023	0.869±0.026	0.904±0.030	0.003±0.000	0.004±0.000	0.033±0.002	8.000±1.000
16	0.566±0.137	0.909±0.021	0.943±0.015	0.487±0.175	0.905±0.022	0.942±0.016	0.935±0.017	0.842±0.034	0.900±0.026	0.003±0.001	0.004±0.001	0.037±0.002	8.000±1.000
17	0.839±0.056	0.825±0.034	0.842±0.030	0.837±0.058	0.817±0.038	0.836±0.034	0.855±0.045	0.795±0.039	0.816±0.035	0.004±0.001	0.005±0.001	0.042±0.006	7.000±1.000
18	0.800±0.045	0.799±0.066	0.806±0.069	0.792±0.048	0.796±0.068	0.803±0.072	0.837±0.037	0.786±0.069	0.786±0.070	0.004±0.000	0.004±0.000	0.041±0.003	8.000±1.000
19	0.331±0.235	0.910±0.015	0.936±0.025	0.257±0.192	0.906±0.017	0.933±0.027	0.933±0.008	0.842±0.026	0.886±0.043	0.004±0.001	0.005±0.000	0.040±0.003	8.000±0.000
20	1.000±0.000	0.985±0.010	0.991±0.008	1.000±0.000	0.985±0.010	0.991±0.008	1.000±0.000	0.971±0.018	0.983±0.016	0.004±0.001	0.005±0.000	0.038±0.002	7.000±0.000
21	1.000±0.000	0.988±0.010	0.993±0.006	1.000±0.000	0.988±0.010	0.993±0.006	1.000±0.000	0.978±0.019	0.986±0.012	0.004±0.001	0.005±0.001	0.038±0.007	7.000±0.000
22	0.974±0.033	0.999±0.003	1.000±0.000	0.973±0.034	0.999±0.003	1.000±0.000	0.994±0.008	0.998±0.005	1.000±0.000	0.004±0.001	0.005±0.001	0.030±0.001	6.000±0.000
23	0.954±0.016	0.993±0.006	0.993±0.006	0.953±0.017	0.993±0.006	0.993±0.006	0.986±0.005	0.989±0.011	0.989±0.011	0.004±0.001	0.004±0.000	0.031±0.004	6.000±0.000
24	1.000±0.000	0.991±0.004	0.994±0.005	1.000±0.000	0.990±0.004	0.994±0.005	1.000±0.000	0.982±0.008	0.989±0.009	0.007±0.001	0.012±0.002	0.088±0.012	7.000±0.000
25	0.839±0.018	0.896±0.020	0.919±0.010	0.827±0.020	0.895±0.020	0.919±0.010	0.965±0.004	0.936±0.004	0.935±0.006	0.080±0.002	0.614±0.028	5.188±0.995	9.000±2.000
26	0.763±0.036	0.761±0.026	0.782±0.026	0.750±0.043	0.761±0.026	0.782±0.026	0.815±0.021	0.761±0.022	0.780±0.026	0.021±0.001	0.057±0.001	0.224±0.037	9.000±2.000
27	0.536±0.121	0.980±0.003	0.987±0.003	0.446±0.155	0.980±0.003	0.987±0.003	0.992±0.002	0.960±0.006	0.974±0.006	0.033±0.001	0.122±0.003	0.454±0.028	8.000±1.000
28	0.992±0.005	0.992±0.006	0.993±0.005	0.992±0.006	0.992±0.006	0.993±0.005	0.998±0.002	0.996±0.002	0.997±0.002	0.049±0.001	0.226±0.015	0.869±0.081	7.000±1.000
29	0.932±0.054	0.999±0.000	0.999±0.000	0.929±0.058	0.999±0.000	0.999±0.000	0.998±0.001	0.999±0.001	0.999±0.001	0.012±0.001	0.026±0.002	1.490±0.119	6.000±1.000
30	0.997±0.006	0.986±0.004	0.989±0.005	0.997±0.006	0.986±0.005	0.989±0.005	0.998±0.003	0.979±0.007	0.983±0.007	0.012±0.001	0.026±0.002	0.204±0.011	6.000±1.000
31	0.847±0.019	0.844±0.026	0.860±0.025	0.842±0.020	0.839±0.028	0.857±0.025	0.894±0.010	0.805±0.030	0.827±0.026	0.012±0.000	0.026±0.001	0.219±0.017	8.000±1.000
32	0.835±0.036	0.825±0.012	0.847±0.020	0.828±0.040	0.815±0.013	0.841±0.018	0.892±0.018	0.771±0.015	0.807±0.014	0.010±0.001	0.026±0.001	0.228±0.020	9.000±1.000
33	0.346±0.298	0.969±0.005	0.975±0.005	0.300±0.258	0.969±0.005	0.975±0.005	0.988±0.002	0.940±0.020	0.951±0.020	0.013±0.001	0.020±0.000	0.165±0.012	9.000±1.000
34	0.129±0.136	0.851±0.033	0.874±0.030	0.063±0.066	0.849±0.031	0.872±0.029	0.970±0.001	0.803±0.014	0.823±0.012	0.022±0.001	0.065±0.001	0.677±0.111	10.000±2.000
35	0.000±0.000	0.915±0.018	0.936±0.011	0.000±0.000	0.912±0.011	0.933±0.012	0.980±0.000	0.841±0.019	0.878±0.018	0.012±0.000	0.026±0.001	0.224±0.018	13.000±2.000
36	0.338±0.309	0.936±0.016	0.953±0.012	0.289±0.281	0.934±0.017	0.952±0.013	0.980±0.005	0.879±0.029	0.910±0.023	0.009±0.000	0.019±0.001	0.151±0.009	8.000±1.000
37	0.608±0.224	0.904±0.048	0.942±0.039	0.563±0.216	0.903±0.049	0.941±0.040	0.991±0.003	0.925±0.010	0.942±0.011	0.020±0.001	0.058±0.001	0.775±0.189	14.000±4.000
38	0.843±0.080	0.947±0.040	0.970±0.010	0.828±0.090	0.947±0.040	0.970±0.011	0.994±0.003	0.930±0.017	0.943±0.020	0.013±0.001	0.028±0.001	0.229±0.016	8.000±1.000
39	0.674±0.071	0.820±0.033	0.830±0.029	0.625±0.091	0.816±0.035	0.827±0.031	0.941±0.010	0.885±0.016	0.891±0.016	0.014±0.001	0.032±0.001	0.401±0.065	13.000±3.000
40	0.887±0.020	0.924±0.017	0.924±0.017	0.881±0.022	0.923±0.017	0.924±0.018	0.976±0.004	0.950±0.006	0.951±0.007	0.014±0.001	0.032±0.001	0.247±0.038	7.000±1.000
41	0.479±0.134	0.713±0.058	0.743±0.057	0.380±0.164	0.707±0.064	0.736±0.062	0.923±0.015	0.775±0.024	0.829±0.030	0.007±0.000	0.012±0.000	0.186±0.054	15.000±4.000
42	0.699±0.096	0.878±0.033	0.899±0.030	0.655±0.121	0.877±0.033	0.898±0.030	0.946±0.016	0.877±0.025	0.894±0.028	0.007±0.000	0.013±0.000	0.124±0.025	9.000±2.000
43	0.261±0.188	0.791±0.099	0.832±0.069	0.173±0.136	0.786±0.105	0.829±0.070	0.970±0.003	0.812±0.003	0.835±0.025	0.013±0.001	0.030±0.002	0.291±0.024	10.000±1.000
44	0.133±0.172	0.763±0.051	0.812±0.051	0.080±0.103	0.758±0.047	0.809±0.050	0.958±0.002	0.710±0.030	0.776±0.023	0.010±0.001	0.020±0.001	0.273±0.069	13.000±3.000
45	0.659±0.107	0.826±0.046	0.856±0.044	0.604±0.136	0.822±0.052	0.855±0.045	0.964±0.009	0.823±0.023	0.840±0.024	0.006±0.000	0.011±0.001	0.114±0.016	10.000±1.000
46	0.870±0.051	0.958±0.018	0.971±0.021	0.861±0.057	0.958±0.018	0.971±0.021	0.976±0.009	0.961±0.011	0.970±0.013	0.007±0.000	0.012±0.001	0.104±0.012	9.000±1.000
47	0.839±0.115	0.875±0.056	0.884±0.065	0.822±0.139	0.869±0.062	0.880±0.067	0.988±0.007	0.953±0.011	0.938±0.061	0.007±0.001	0.011±0.001	0.104±0.018	8.000±1.000
48	0.418±0.113	0.831±0.021	0.867±0.025	0.305±0.134	0.831±0.022	0.867±0.025	0.971±0.004	0.856±0.012	0.875±0.011	0.021±0.001	0.060±0.004	0.595±0.132	10.000±2.000
49	0.635±0.107	0.969±0.005	0.973±0.005	0.574±0.136	0.969±0.005	0.972±0.005	0.980±0.004	0.941±0.009	0.947±0.010	0.020±0.001	0.059±0.009	0.429±0.009	7.000±0.000
50	0.591±0.107	0.893±0.035	0.924±0.025	0.520±0.133	0.892±0.036	0.923±0.025	0.985±0.002	0.916±0.011	0.918±0.017	0.020±0.001	0.060±0.003	0.793±0.332	14.000±6.000

Table 3. The comparative results among UnWELM, WELM, and SawELM with $(C, L) = (2^{20}, 500)$

Data set	Testing G-mean			Testing F-measure			Testing accuracy			Training time			Iterations
	UnWELM	WELM	SawELM	UnWELM	WELM	SawELM	UnWELM	WELM	SawELM	UnWELM	WELM	SawELM	
1	0.883±0.151	0.966±0.012	0.970±0.010	0.867±0.172	0.865±0.012	0.970±0.010	0.995±0.006	0.935±0.022	0.943±0.018	0.014±0.001	0.020±0.001	0.155±0.007	7.000±0.000
2	0.928±0.072	0.992±0.007	0.997±0.003	0.924±0.078	0.992±0.007	0.997±0.003	0.990±0.009	0.986±0.012	0.995±0.006	0.014±0.001	0.020±0.001	0.171±0.013	8.000±0.000
3	0.897±0.092	0.946±0.047	0.957±0.048	0.888±0.105	0.944±0.049	0.956±0.050	0.985±0.013	0.965±0.017	0.964±0.016	0.015±0.001	0.023±0.001	0.193±0.020	8.000±1.000
4	0.932±0.057	0.984±0.022	0.990±0.006	0.928±0.061	0.984±0.022	0.990±0.006	0.991±0.007	0.984±0.012	0.981±0.011	0.015±0.000	0.023±0.001	0.196±0.004	8.000±0.000
5	0.974±0.042	0.987±0.008	0.990±0.007	0.973±0.044	0.987±0.008	0.990±0.006	0.995±0.008	0.977±0.014	0.982±0.012	0.011±0.001	0.016±0.003	0.127±0.016	7.000±0.000
6	0.974±0.042	0.964±0.039	0.987±0.011	0.973±0.044	0.963±0.041	0.987±0.011	0.995±0.007	0.977±0.013	0.977±0.019	0.012±0.002	0.018±0.004	0.157±0.020	8.000±0.000
7	1.000±0.000	0.990±0.007	0.993±0.006	1.000±0.000	0.990±0.007	0.993±0.006	1.000±0.000	0.982±0.012	0.987±0.010	0.012±0.002	0.017±0.002	0.133±0.018	7.000±0.000
8	0.931±0.071	0.950±0.052	0.991±0.005	0.927±0.079	0.948±0.055	0.990±0.005	0.988±0.012	0.983±0.011	0.983±0.009	0.012±0.001	0.018±0.001	0.150±0.009	8.000±1.000
9	1.000±0.000	0.997±0.004	0.997±0.004	1.000±0.000	0.995±0.005	0.997±0.005	0.997±0.007	0.992±0.009	0.995±0.008	0.011±0.001	0.015±0.000	0.121±0.009	7.000±0.000
10	1.000±0.000	0.994±0.007	0.994±0.007	1.000±0.000	0.989±0.009	0.994±0.007	1.000±0.000	0.980±0.015	0.990±0.012	0.019±0.026	0.017±0.003	0.125±0.015	7.000±0.000
11	0.939±0.042	0.928±0.042	0.987±0.008	0.936±0.044	0.926±0.044	0.986±0.008	0.989±0.007	0.968±0.015	0.976±0.015	0.012±0.001	0.016±0.001	0.153±0.010	9.000±1.000
12	0.819±0.060	0.946±0.004	0.946±0.005	0.805±0.070	0.944±0.004	0.945±0.005	0.949±0.012	0.905±0.007	0.906±0.008	0.012±0.001	0.023±0.001	0.188±0.013	8.000±0.000
13	0.999±0.003	0.976±0.015	0.983±0.015	0.999±0.003	0.975±0.016	0.983±0.015	0.998±0.005	0.963±0.023	0.975±0.023	0.012±0.001	0.016±0.001	0.135±0.009	8.000±1.00
14	0.383±0.351	0.915±0.016	0.943±0.020	0.348±0.336	0.911±0.017	0.941±0.021	0.933±0.022	0.851±0.026	0.898±0.034	0.011±0.000	0.016±0.000	0.141±0.008	8.000±0.000
15	0.765±0.118	0.932±0.021	0.949±0.018	0.734±0.139	0.930±0.022	0.947±0.019	0.957±0.020	0.882±0.035	0.910±0.031	0.010±0.000	0.014±0.000	0.111±0.005	7.000±0.000
16	0.720±0.126	0.927±0.027	0.942±0.021	0.681±0.152	0.924±0.029	0.941±0.022	0.946±0.025	0.872±0.045	0.898±0.036	0.010±0.001	0.015±0.001	0.128±0.011	8.000±1.000
17	0.828±0.025	0.841±0.033	0.847±0.029	0.826±0.026	0.836±0.035	0.842±0.031	0.852±0.025	0.817±0.038	0.823±0.039	0.010±0.000	0.016±0.000	0.128±0.011	7.000±0.000
18	0.805±0.054	0.782±0.044	0.808±0.035	0.797±0.061	0.778±0.045	0.805±0.036	0.841±0.033	0.767±0.048	0.790±0.040	0.011±0.001	0.016±0.000	0.163±0.015	9.000±1.000
19	0.585±0.130	0.918±0.025	0.934±0.021	0.511±0.167	0.914±0.027	0.932±0.023	0.945±0.011	0.855±0.042	0.883±0.037	0.011±0.001	0.016±0.001	0.141±0.011	8.000±0.000
20	1.000±0.000	0.982±0.007	0.984±0.008	1.000±0.000	0.982±0.008	0.984±0.008	1.000±0.000	0.967±0.014	0.970±0.014	0.011±0.001	0.017±0.001	0.126±0.004	7.000±0.000
21	1.000±0.000	0.989±0.000	0.993±0.006	1.000±0.000	0.989±0.000	0.993±0.006	1.000±0.000	0.979±0.015	0.986±0.012	0.011±0.001	0.016±0.001	0.119±0.008	7.000±0.000
22	0.994±0.020	0.998±0.004	1.000±0.000	0.993±0.021	0.998±0.004	1.000±0.000	0.998±0.005	0.997±0.007	1.000±0.000	0.011±0.000	0.016±0.001	0.115±0.008	7.000±0.000
23	0.954±0.030	0.996±0.005	0.997±0.004	0.952±0.031	0.996±0.005	0.997±0.005	0.986±0.009	0.994±0.008	0.995±0.008	0.011±0.001	0.016±0.001	0.111±0.008	6.000±0.000
24	1.000±0.000	0.991±0.007	0.994±0.005	1.000±0.000	0.991±0.007	0.994±0.005	1.000±0.000	0.983±0.013	0.988±0.009	0.019±0.001	0.032±0.001	0.249±0.004	7.000±0.000
25	0.851±0.026	0.907±0.013	0.924±0.010	0.841±0.029	0.907±0.014	0.924±0.010	0.965±0.005	0.932±0.006	0.935±0.006	0.199±0.008	1.115±0.061	9.808±1.672	6.000±2.000
26	0.758±0.029	0.770±0.028	0.792±0.027	0.743±0.035	0.770±0.028	0.792±0.023	0.818±0.018	0.773±0.025	0.792±0.023	0.029±0.002	0.058±0.003	0.576±0.069	10.000±1.000
27	0.730±0.091	0.984±0.004	0.991±0.002	0.692±0.112	0.984±0.004	0.991±0.002	0.995±0.002	0.969±0.008	0.982±0.004	0.055±0.003	0.141±0.007	1.114±0.064	8.000±1.000
28	0.990±0.005	0.993±0.005	0.993±0.005	0.990±0.005	0.993±0.005	0.993±0.005	0.997±0.002	0.997±0.002	0.997±0.002	0.085±0.003	0.253±0.04	1.738±0.103	6.000±0.000
29	0.940±0.046	0.999±0.000	0.999±0.000	0.937±0.049	0.999±0.000	0.999±0.000	0.998±0.001	0.998±0.001	0.999±0.001	0.127±0.012	0.483±0.035	3.532±0.175	7.000±0.000
30	0.998±0.003	0.991±0.004	0.999±0.002	0.998±0.003	0.991±0.004	0.999±0.002	0.998±0.002	0.987±0.006	0.997±0.002	0.033±0.002	0.064±0.002	0.497±0.020	7.000±0.000
31	0.890±0.033	0.860±0.021	0.879±0.023	0.886±0.035	0.854±0.022	0.876±0.024	0.926±0.019	0.819±0.025	0.849±0.026	0.034±0.003	0.067±0.006	0.574±0.034	8.000±1.000
32	0.898±0.024	0.842±0.017	0.871±0.012	0.896±0.026	0.836±0.017	0.868±0.012	0.924±0.011	0.797±0.019	0.840±0.011	0.032±0.002	0.064±0.001	0.595±0.046	9.000±1.000
33	0.534±0.302	0.975±0.006	0.981±0.003	0.490±0.292	0.975±0.006	0.981±0.003	0.991±0.004	0.951±0.011	0.964±0.007	0.026±0.001	0.050±0.003	0.401±0.033	8.000±1.000
34	0.221±0.165	0.869±0.039	0.892±0.027	0.130±0.113	0.867±0.037	0.890±0.026	0.971±0.002	0.820±0.016	0.844±0.016	0.059±0.001	0.155±0.007	1.850±0.321	12.000±2.000
35	0.350±0.253	0.924±0.008	0.939±0.007	0.281±0.216	0.922±0.009	0.937±0.007	0.984±0.003	0.857±0.015	0.883±0.013	0.032±0.001	0.063±0.001	0.563±0.030	8.000±1.000
36	0.654±0.115	0.946±0.010	0.961±0.008	0.597±0.142	0.945±0.011	0.961±0.006	0.986±0.004	0.898±0.019	0.926±0.011	0.026±0.001	0.046±0.000	0.360±0.013	7.000±0.000
37	0.762±0.070	0.909±0.062	0.937±0.053	0.734±0.085	0.907±0.064	0.936±0.055	0.993±0.002	0.922±0.014	0.948±0.006	0.061±0.019	0.143±0.013	2.203±0.297	16.000±2.000
38	0.808±0.124	0.966±0.028	0.983±0.005	0.785±0.149	0.966±0.028	0.983±0.005	0.993±0.004	0.951±0.009	0.967±0.009	0.034±0.001	0.069±0.002	0.579±0.055	8.000±1.000
39	0.710±0.046	0.816±0.039	0.831±0.044	0.672±0.058	0.812±0.042	0.828±0.047	0.946±0.006	0.870±0.012	0.887±0.015	0.037±0.001	0.079±0.001	1.234±0.135	15.000±2.000
40	0.893±0.029	0.930±0.018	0.930±0.018	0.887±0.032	0.929±0.019	0.930±0.018	0.978±0.005	0.955±0.008	0.956±0.008	0.037±0.002	0.079±0.001	0.591±0.099	7.000±0.000
41	0.541±0.147	0.756±0.086	0.803±0.082	0.457±0.181	0.753±0.090	0.798±0.090	0.928±0.017	0.771±0.029	0.846±0.029	0.020±0.000	0.035±0.000	0.614±0.079	17.000±2.000
42	0.733±0.082	0.862±0.043	0.892±0.031	0.699±0.103	0.861±0.045	0.891±0.031	0.953±0.011	0.882±0.021	0.876±0.020	0.022±0.002	0.037±0.001	0.287±0.012	7.000±0.000
43	0.319±0.188	0.808±0.054	0.866±0.038	0.223±0.156	0.807±0.054	0.865±0.037	0.972±0.004	0.819±0.022	0.846±0.023	0.036±0.002	0.074±0.002	0.769±0.101	10.000±1.000
44	0.033±0.105	0.782±0.055	0.824±0.058	0.020±0.063	0.776±0.052	0.821±0.056	0.957±0.002	0.714±0.029	0.781±0.031	0.026±0.001	0.031±0.000	0.658±0.075	13.000±1.000
45	0.620±0.067	0.813±0.082	0.858±0.047	0.556±0.087	0.810±0.086	0.856±0.046	0.960±0.005	0.821±0.029	0.854±0.027	0.019±0.000	0.031±0.000	0.315±0.055	9.000±2.000
46	0.875±0.053	0.951±0.027	0.962±0.023	0.867±0.059	0.951±0.027	0.961±0.023	0.973±0.011	0.961±0.013	0.963±0.011	0.021±0.001	0.036±0.000	0.275±0.003	7.000±0.000
47	0.732±0.126	0.792±0.068	0.871±0.091	0.695±0.158	0.778±0.079	0.862±0.012	0.981±0.007	0.935±0.017	0.970±0.011	0.019±0.000	0.033±0.001	0.424±0.023	12.000±1.000
48	0.417±0.084	0.863±0.031	0.891±0.026	0.300±0.099	0.862±0.031	0.890±0.026	0.972±0.003	0.866±0.011	0.883±0.011	0.055±0.002	0.137±0.003	1.731±0.294	12.000±2.000
49	0.589±0.076	0.966±0.007	0.972±0.005	0.516±0.097	0.965±0.007	0.972±0.005	0.977±0.004	0.935±0.012	0.947±0.010	0.056±0.003	0.138±0.004	1.061±0.018	7.000±0.000
50	0.613±0.063	0.917±0.037	0.917±0.037	0.546±0.082	0.916±0.037	0.916±0.037	0.984±0.002	0.915±0.014	0.916±0.014	0.054±0.001	0.138±0.004	1.170±0.148	8.000±1.000

If $TN_{\text{WELM}} < TN_{\text{SawELM}}$, we can get G-mean$_{\text{WELM}}$ < G-mean$_{\text{SawELM}}s$. Let G-mean$_{\text{WELM}}$ and F-measures$_{\text{SawELM}}$ denote the testing F-measures of WELM and SawELM, where

$$\text{F-measure}_{\text{WELM}} = \frac{2TP}{2TP + FN + FP_{\text{WELM}}}$$

and

$$\text{F-measure}_{\text{SawELM}} = \frac{2TP}{2TP + FN + FP_{\text{SawELM}}}.$$

If $FP_{\text{WELM}} > FP_{\text{SawELM}}$, we can derive F-measure$_{\text{WELM}}$ < F-measure$_{\text{SawELM}}$. In addition, Tables 2 and 3 show that the training time of SawELM is higher than UnWELM and WELM. This is because SawELM requires the necessary iterations to adjust the instance weights and update the instance outputs.

5   Conclusions and Further Works

In this paper, we proposed an improved version of weighted extreme learning machine (WELM), i.e., self-adaptive WELM (SawELM) which further enhanced the imbalanced classification capability of WELM by gradually reducing the weights of wrongly-classified training instances and dynamically updating the outputs of wrongly-classified instances. The final experiments demonstrated that SawELM obtained the obviously better testing G-mean, testing F-measure, and testing accuracy than WELM. Our future works include the following two topics. Firstly, we will try to improve the stability of SawELM with Gaussian process regression. Secondly, we will extend SawELM into the scenario of imbalanced multi-class classification problems.

Acknowledgments. The first author and second author contributed equally the same to this article which is supported by National Natural Science Foundations of China (61503252 and 61473194) and China Postdoctoral Science Foundation (2016T90799).

References

1. Alcalá-Fdez, J., Sánchez, L., García, S., del Jesus, M.J., Ventura, S., Garrell, J.M., Otero, J., Romero, C., Bacardit, J., Rivas, V.M., Fernández, J.C., Herrera, F.: KEEL: a software tool to assess evolutionary algorithms to data mining problems. Soft. Comput. **13**(3), 307–318 (2009)
2. Alcalá-Fdez, J., Fernandez, A., Luengo, J., Derrac, J., García, S., Sánchez, L., Herrera, F.: KEEL data-mining software tool: data set repository. Integration of algorithms and experimental analysis framework. J. Multiple-Valued Logic Soft Comput. **17**(2–3), 255–287 (2011)
3. Ertekin, S., Huang, J., Bottou, L., Giles, C.L.: Learning on the border: active learning in imbalanced data classification. In: Proceedings of the Sixteenth ACM Conference on Information and Knowledge Management, pp. 127–136 (2007)

4. Ertekin, S., Huang, J., Giles, C.L.: Active learning for class imbalance problem. In: Proceedings of The 30th Annual International ACM SIGIR Conference on Research and Development in Information Retrieval, pp. 823–824 (2007)

5. Guo, H., Viktor, H.L.: Learning from imbalanced data sets with boosting and data generation: the databoost-im approach. ACM SIGKDD Explor. Newslett. **6**(1), 30–39 (2004)

6. Han, H., Wang, W.-Y., Mao, B.-H.: Borderline-SMOTE: a new over-sampling method in imbalanced data sets learning. In: Huang, D.-S., Zhang, X.-P., Huang, G.-B. (eds.) ICIC 2005. LNCS, vol. 3644, pp. 878–887. Springer, Heidelberg (2005). doi:10.1007/11538059_91

7. He, H.B., Garcia, E.A.: Learning from imbalanced data. IEEE Trans. Knowl. Data Eng. **21**(9), 1263–1284 (2009)

8. He, H.B., Ma, Y.Q.: Imbalanced Learning: Foundations, Algorithms, and Applications. Wiley, Hoboken (2013)

9. Huang, G.B., Zhou, H., Ding, X., Zhang, R.: Extreme learning machine for regression and multiclass classification. IEEE Trans. Syst. Man Cybern. B Cybern. **42**(2), 513–529 (2012)

10. Huang, G.B., Zhu, Q.Y., Siew, C.K.: Extreme learning machine: theory and applications. Neurocomputing **70**(1), 489–501 (2006)

11. Khoshgoftaar, T.M., Van Hulse, J., Napolitano, A.: Comparing boosting and bagging techniques with noisy and imbalanced data. IEEE Trans. Syst. Man Cybern. Part A Syst. Hum. **41**(3), 552–568 (2011)

12. Li, K., Kong, X.F., Lu, Z., Liu, W.Y., Yin, J.P.: Boosting weighted ELM for imbalanced learning. Neurocomputing **128**, 15–21 (2014)

13. Liu, X.Y., Wu, J.X., Zhou, Z.H.: Exploratory undersampling for class-imbalance learning. IEEE Trans. Syst. Man Cybern. B Cybern. **39**(2), 539–550 (2009)

14. Thai-Nghe, N., Gantner, Z., Schmidt-Thieme, L.: Cost-sensitive learning methods for imbalanced data. In: Proceedings of the 2010 International Joint Conference on Neural Networks, pp. 1–8 (2010)

15. Xiao, W.D., Zhang, J., Li, Y.J., Yang, W.D.: Imbalanced extreme learning machine for classification with imbalanced data distributions. Proc. Adapt. Learn. Optimization **7**, 503–514 (2016)

16. Yang, J., Yu, H., Yang, X., Zuo, X.: Imbalanced extreme learning machine based on probability density estimation. In: Bikakis, A., Zheng, X. (eds.) MIWAI 2015. LNCS, vol. 9426, pp. 160–167. Springer, Cham (2015). doi:10.1007/978-3-319-26181-2_15

17. You, Z.H., Lei, Y.K., Zhu, L., Xia, J.F., Wang, B.: Prediction of protein-protein interactions from amino acid sequences with ensemble extreme learning machines and principal component analysis. BMC Bioinform. **14**(Suppl 8), S10 (2013)

18. Zadrozny, B., Langford, J., Abe, N.: Cost-sensitive learning by cost-proportionate example weighting. In: Proceedings of the Third IEEE International Conference on Data Mining, pp. 435–442 (2003)

19. Zhang, S., Qin, Z., Ling, C.X., Sheng, S.: "Missing is useful": missing values in cost-sensitive decision trees. IEEE Trans. Knowl. Data Eng. **17**(12), 1689–1693 (2005)

20. Zhou, Z.H., Liu, X.Y.: Training cost-sensitive neural networks with methods addressing the class imbalance problem. IEEE Trans. Knowl. Data Eng. **18**(1), 63–77 (2006)

21. Zong, W.W., Huang, G.B., Chen, Y.Q.: Weighted extreme learning machine for imbalance learning. Neurocomputing **101**, 229–242 (2013)

Estimating Word Probabilities with Neural Networks in Latent Dirichlet Allocation

Tomonari Masada[✉]

Nagasaki University, 1-14 Bunkyo-machi, Nagasaki 8528521, Japan
masada@nagasaki-u.ac.jp

Abstract. This paper proposes a new method for estimating the word probabilities in latent Dirichlet allocation (LDA). LDA uses a Dirichlet distribution as the prior for the per-document topic discrete distributions. While another Dirichlet prior can be introduced for the per-topic word discrete distributions, point estimations may lead to a better evaluation result, e.g. in terms of test perplexity. This paper proposes a method for the point estimation of the per-topic word probabilities in LDA by using multilayer perceptron (MLP). Our point estimation is performed in an online manner by mini-batch gradient ascent. We compared our method to the baseline method using a perceptron with no hidden layers and also to the collapsed Gibbs sampling (CGS). The evaluation experiment showed that the test perplexity of CGS could not be improved in almost all cases. However, there certainly were situations where our method achieved a better perplexity than the baseline. We also discuss a usage of our method as word embedding.

1 Introduction

Topic modeling [3,6] is widely used for obtaining a lower-dimensional representation of documents and has many interdisciplinary applications [4,7,9]. Intuitively, topic models are proposed based on the observation that we use different sets of vocabulary for talking about different things. The bag-of-words model represents documents as vectors of dimension V, where V is the number of different words appearing in the corpus. By using latent Dirichlet allocation (LDA) [3], the best known topic model, we can reduce the dimension of the document representation space from V to K, where K is the number of latent topics. This reduction is achieved by representing each document as a mixture of K latent topics, where the mixture proportions give a lower-dimensional representation of each document. Each of the K latent topics is, in turn, modeled as a discrete distribution defined over words. Therefore, we can make a word list by picking up the words having large probabilities in each of the K word probability distributions. Such word lists may give useful and intuitive hints on what kind of things are talked about in the given corpus (cf. Fig. 1).

This paper proposes a new method for estimating the parameters of the per-topic word discrete distributions in LDA. LDA uses a Dirichlet distribution as the prior distribution for the per-document topic discrete distributions. This is

© Springer International Publishing AG 2017
U Kang et al. (Eds.): PAKDD 2017 Workshops, LNAI 10526, pp. 129–137, 2017.
DOI: 10.1007/978-3-319-67274-8_12

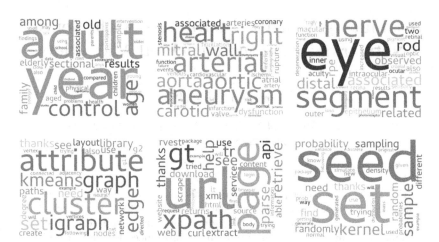

Fig. 1. Word lists obtained by our method from the MEDLINE data set (top) and from the Stack Overflow data set (bottom). Each list corresponds to a different topic.

the reason why the method is called "latent Dirichlet" allocation. We can also introduce another Dirichlet prior for the per-topic word discrete distributions. However, point estimations may lead to a better evaluation result, e.g. in terms of test perplexity. In fact, the original paper [3] performs a point estimation for the per-topic word probabilities. Our method also performs a point estimation of the per-topic word probabilities. The estimation is implemented as an online one by mini-batch gradient ascent. The main contribution of this paper is to modify the online inference for LDA [8] by using multilayer perceptron (MLP) toward a better point estimation of the per-topic word probabilities.

The input layer of MLP used by our method consists of K nodes. The input vector is a K-dimensional one-hot vector representing one among the K topics. The output layer consists of V nodes. The output vector is converted into a word probability distribution with the softmax function. We only consider MLP with a single hidden layer of size M. The input and the hidden layers are fully connected, and the hidden and the output layers are also fully connected. The baseline method for the comparison experiment uses the perceptron having no hidden layers. The experimental results showed that there certainly were situations where the proposed method achieved a better test perplexity than the baseline. We also compared our method to the collapsed Gibbs sampling (CGS) for LDA [6]. Our method could not improve CGS for almost all cases. However, the online inference has an advantage in memory consumption when compared to CGS.

Additionally, it will be discussed that our method may work as a word embedding, which is what the vanilla LDA cannot achieve. The network weights between the hidden and the output layers can be regarded as the coordinates of the M-dimensional word embedding. This embedding is corpus-wide, where

M can be chosen regardless of K. We will show an example of the similar word pairs obtained by computing the Euclidean distance in the embedding space.

2 Related Work

Miao et al. [11] have proposed a document model called neural variational document model (NVDM). NVDM uses a neural network to encode each document as a lower-dimensional latent vector, whose entries are the parameters of the diagonal multivariate normal distribution. Then the decoder network converts samples from the normal distribution into word probability distributions. NVDM greatly improves LDA in terms of test perplexity. However, the per-document latent vectors have no intuitive interpretation. In contrast, the per-document topic probabilities in LDA can be interpreted as the relevance of the topics in each document. Further, NVDM gives as many word probability distributions as documents. In contrast, LDA provides a fixed number of word probability distributions, each of which corresponds to a distinct latent topic. Therefore, those word probability distributions can be regarded as an intuitive summary of the corpus (cf. Fig. 1). We only modify the estimation method of the per-topic word probabilities in LDA. Therefore, the results given by our method are as easy to interpret as those given by LDA.

Srivastava et al. [14] have proposed a method to use neural networks in the inference for topic models. Their method, named ProdLDA, follows the proposal of Kingma et al. [10] and adopts the reparameterization trick for the variational posterior distribution, whose parameters are the outputs of a feedforward neural network. The expectation appearing in the lower bound of the log evidence is estimated by using the samples from the approximate posterior. On the other hand, our method performs the original variational Bayesian inference described in [3] and only modifies the way the per-topic word probabilities are estimated. Therefore, an additional complication for the estimation of the word probabilities introduced by ProdLDA is not required for our method.

3 Method

3.1 Latent Dirichlet Allocation

Let D denote the number of documents and N_d the length, i.e., the number of word tokens, of the dth document. Let V be the vocabulary size, i.e., the number of different words. We write the event that the ith word token of the dth document is the vth word as $x_{d,i} = v$. The $x_{d,i}$s are observable variables. Let K be the number of topics. For each word token $x_{d,i}$, we have a latent variable $z_{d,i}$ giving its topic assignment. We write the event that the ith word token of the dth document is assigned to the kth topic as $z_{d,i} = k$. Latent Dirichlet allocation (LDA) [3] generates a corpus as below.

1. For $d = 1, \ldots, D$, draw a per-document topic probability distribution $\boldsymbol{\theta}_d = (\theta_{d,1}, \ldots, \theta_{d,K})$ from the Dirichlet prior distribution $\texttt{Dirichlet}(\alpha)$. $\theta_{d,k}$ is the probability that the word tokens of the dth document are assigned to the kth topic. In this paper, we only consider the symmetric Dirichlet prior.
   (a) For $i = 1, \ldots, N_d$, draw a topic from the per-document topic discrete distribution $\texttt{Discrete}(\boldsymbol{\theta}_d)$ and set the value of $z_{d,i}$ to the drawn topic.
   (b) For $i = 1, \ldots, N_d$, draw a word from the word discrete distribution $\texttt{Discrete}(\boldsymbol{\phi}_{z_{d,i}})$ corresponding to the drawn topic $z_{d,i}$ and set the value of $x_{d,i}$ to the drawn word. Here, $\boldsymbol{\phi}_k = (\phi_{k,1}, \ldots, \phi_{k,V})$ denotes the parameter of the word discrete distribution for the kth topic. That is, $\phi_{k,v}$ denotes the probability of the vth word in the kth topic.

It can be said that LDA gives a clustering of the word tokens based on their topic assignments. The latent variable $z_{d,i}$ tells to which topic the ith word token of the dth document is assigned. The word tokens assigned to the same topic are expected to express a similar *topic* in the ordinary sense of this word.

In this paper, we adopt the variational Bayesian inference for the estimation of the posterior parameters of LDA. We obtain a lower bound of the log evidence of the dth document as below [3].

$$\log p(\boldsymbol{x}_d; \alpha, \boldsymbol{\Phi}) \geq \sum_{i=1}^{N_d} \sum_{k=1}^{K} \gamma_{d,i,k} \log \phi_{k,x_{d,i}}$$
$$+ \sum_{k=1}^{K} \left(\alpha + \sum_{i=1}^{N_d} \gamma_{d,i,k} - \eta_{d,k} \right) \left\{ \Psi(\eta_{d,k}) - \Psi\left(\sum_{k'=1}^{K} \eta_{d,k'} \right) \right\}$$
$$- \sum_{i=1}^{N_d} \sum_{k=1}^{K} \gamma_{d,i,k} \log \gamma_{d,i,k} + \log \Gamma(K\alpha) - K \log \Gamma(\alpha) \qquad (1)$$

The parameters are estimated by maximizing the lower bound in Eq. (1). $\gamma_{d,i,k}$ is the variational approximate probability that the ith word token of the dth document is assigned to the kth topic, satisfying $\sum_{k=1}^{K} \gamma_{d,i,k} = 1$. The $\eta_{d,k}$s are the parameters of the variational Dirichlet posterior for the per-document topic discrete distributions. By differentiating the lower bound in Eq. (1) with respect to $\eta_{d,k}$ and $\gamma_{d,i,k}$, we obtain the formulas $\eta_{d,k} \leftarrow \alpha + \sum_{i=1}^{N_d} \gamma_{d,i,k}$ and $\gamma_{d,i,k} \leftarrow \propto \phi_{k,x_{d,i}} \times \frac{\exp\{\Psi(\eta_{d,k})\}}{\exp\{\Psi(\sum_k \eta_{d,k})\}}$ for the coordinate ascent update.

3.2 Online Estimation of Word Probabilities with MLP

We propose a new method for updating the per-topic word probabilities $\boldsymbol{\phi}_k$ for $k = 1, \ldots, K$ in Eq. (1). Our method obtains each $\boldsymbol{\phi}_k$ by using multilayer perceptron (MLP). The input layer consists of K nodes, where the one-hot input vector whose kth entry is 1 corresponds to the kth latent topic. Therefore, we only have K different inputs and thus only have K different outputs, which are in turn converted into the per-topic word probability distributions. We denote the V-dimensional output vector for the kth topic as $\boldsymbol{y}_k = (y_{k,1}, \ldots, y_{k,V})$. The parameter $\phi_{k,v}$ is obtained by applying the softmax function to the output, i.e., $\phi_{k,v} = \frac{\exp(y_{k,v})}{\sum_{v'} \exp(y_{k,v'})}$. Only the first term of the lower bound in Eq. (1) contains the $\phi_{k,v}$s. Therefore, we can point-estimate them by maximizing the term.

In this paper, we only consider MLP with a single hidden layer. Let M be the number of hidden layer nodes. The input and the hidden layers are fully connected. We denote the bias of the mth hidden node and the weight between the mth hidden node and the kth input node as $u_{m,0}$ and $u_{m,k}$, respectively. The hidden and the output layers are also fully connected. We denote the bias of the vth output node and the weight between the vth output node and the mth hidden node as $w_{v,0}$ and $w_{v,m}$, respectively. The ReLU [13] activation function $\sigma(\cdot)$ is applied to the hidden layer. Since we use the one-hot input vectors, $y_{k,v} = \sum_{m=1}^{M} w_{v,m} \sigma(u_{m,k} + u_{m,0}) + w_{v,0}$ holds. Let $\sigma(u_{m,k} + u_{m,0})$ be denoted as $t_{m,k}$. Then $y_{k,v} = \sum_{m=0}^{M} w_{v,m} t_{m,k} = \boldsymbol{w}_v \cdot \boldsymbol{t}_k$, where we assume that $t_{0,k} \equiv 1$.

We can take the equation $y_{k,v} = \boldsymbol{w}_v \cdot \boldsymbol{t}_k$ as a factorization under the non-negativity constraint for one among the two factors, because the ReLU is non-negative. This factorization is performed not for the dimensionality reduction but for the embedding. The vector $\boldsymbol{w}_v$ can be regarded as an embedding of the vth word in the $(M + 1)$-dimensional space, where M can be chosen regardless of K. As will be discussed later, $\boldsymbol{w}_v$ can be used for finding similar words.

We compare our method to the baseline, which is the point estimation using the perceptron with no hidden layers. The baseline method also applies the softmax function for obtaining the word probabilities, i.e., $\phi_{k,v} = \frac{\exp(y_{k,v})}{\sum_{v'} \exp(y_{k,v'})}$. Since the input vector is a K-dimensional one-hot vector, the baseline method is equivalent to the direct estimation of the $\phi_{k,v}$s by maximizing the first term of the lower bound in Eq. (1). This estimation by the baseline is also performed in an online manner by mini-batch gradient ascent.

We further compare our method to the collapsed Gibbs sampling (CGS) for LDA [6]. Since CGS is a sampling from the posterior, it is likely to achieve a better evaluation result when compared to the variational Bayesian inference, where an approximation is introduced. However, the variational inference for LDA can easily be performed in an online manner by mini-batch gradient ascent. In contrast, CGS is difficult to operate with a small amount of memory.

4   Experiment

We prepared two corpora for the comparison experiment. The one is a subset of the MEDLINE/PubMed data set[1]. We used the paper abstracts of length less than or equal to 512 contained in the XML files from `medline14n0770.xml` to `medline14n0774.xml` of the annual baseline in 2015. The other is a subset of the questions in the Stack Overflow data set[2] We used the questions of length less than or equal to 256. For both data sets, we reduced the vocabulary size

---

[1] https://www.nlm.nih.gov/databases/download/pubmed_medline.html.
[2] https://www.kaggle.com/stackoverflow/rquestions.

Table 1. Specifications of the two document sets used in our evaluation.

	# documents	# different words	# training (test) word tokens
MEDLINE	64,731	9,166	6,405,672 (637,878)
Stack Overflow	142,850	7,958	9,522,510 (956,410)

by discarding highly-frequent and rare words after converting all words to lower case. The specifications of the two data sets are given in Table 1.

The online parameter estimation by the baseline and our proposed method was performed on mini-batches of size 200. Smaller mini-batches could not improve the results. Adagrad [5] was adopted for the gradient-based optimization, where the learning rate ρ was grid-searched. The dropout [15] was applied to the hidden layer of our method with a probability of 0.5. Further, the layer normalization [2] was applied to the hidden layer. Randomly chosen 90% documents were used for training, and the rest 10% documents were used for computing the test perplexity. We compared the methods in terms of test perplexity, because this is an evaluation measure often used for comparing topic models [1,3].

The results are summarized in Table 2. The following three settings were applied for the number of topics: $K = 64, 128$, and 192. The test perplexities of CGS in Table 2 were obtained by iterating through the training set 3,000 times. We used a grid search with respect to the symmetric Dirichlet hyperparameters α and β [1] for CGS. The test perplexities of the baseline and our method in Table 2 were obtained by looping over the training set 100 times. We set the symmetric Dirichlet parameter α to 0.01 for the baseline and our method.

We implemented the baseline and our method in C/CUDA and ran both methods on NVIDIA GTX970 or GTX1060. Due to a computational resource limitation, we could only test a limited number of settings for the learning rate ρ. The hidden layer size M was set to 512 for all cases. The walk-clock time measured on the MEDLINE data set was around 11 h for CGS when $K = 128$, around 21 h for the baseline when $K = 128$, and around 75 h for our method when $K = 128$ and $M = 512$. However, the running time of the baseline and our method heavily depends on the performance of GPU.

Table 2. Evaluation results in terms of test perplexity

Data set (K)	CGS	Baseline (ρ)	Our method (M, ρ)
MEDLINE (64)	1314.457	1518.995 (0.3)	1500.525 (512, 0.03)
MEDLINE (128)	1077.015	1220.686 (1.0)	1224.791 (512, 0.02)
MEDLINE (192)	944.458	1059.218 (1.1)	1086.717 (512, 0.015)
Stack Overflow (64)	747.367	841.072 (0.7)	833.437 (512, 0.02)
Stack Overflow (128)	600.194	617.725 (0.8)	622.930 (512, 0.02)
Stack Overflow (192)	523.030	508.241 (0.9)	502.985 (512, 0.02)

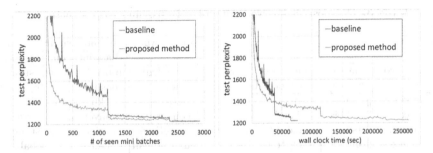

Fig. 2. The above two charts show how the test perplexity decreased as learning proceeded when $K = 128$ for the MEDLINE data. The same evaluation data are depicted
in both panels. But a different unit is used for the horizontal axis. The vertical axis
gives the test perplexity in both panels. The horizontal axis in the left panel gives the
number of seen mini-batches, and that of the right panel gives the wall clock time. Our
method could decrease the test perplexity more rapidly at earlier iterations.

Table 2 shows that the perplexity of CGS was improved only in a single case,
i.e., $K = 192$ for the Stack Overflow data set. The online variational Bayesian
inference seems to work better for a larger number of topics. The underline
in Table 2 shows which was the better between the baseline and our method.
Our method improved the baseline for three cases among six. Therefore, there
certainly were situations where our method achieved a better test perplexity
than the baseline. If a better estimation of the word probabilities, even if only
slightly better, is required, our method can be adopted as an alternative. The
words of large probability obtained by our method are presented as word clouds[3]
in Fig. 1, where an intuitive display of each topic as a word list can be found.

Figure 2 presents how the test perplexity decreased as learning proceeded
when $K = 128$ for the MEDLINE data set. The same evaluation data in terms
of test perplexity are depicted in both of the left and the right panels. However,
a different unit is used for the horizontal axis. The horizontal axis of the chart
on the left panel gives the number of seen mini-batches, and that of the chart on
the right gives the wall clock time. Large drops observable in both charts were
brought about by a scheduled modification of the learning rate ρ. The chart on
the left shows that our method could achieve the same test perplexity with a
smaller number of mini-batches at earlier iterations. Further, the chart on the
right shows that our method gave a smaller perplexity before the first large
drop occurred for the baseline even when the methods were compared in the
real time scale. While the final test perplexity given by our method showed no
large discrepancy from that of the baseline, Fig. 2 provides an advantage of our
method, i.e., a rapid decrease of the test perplexity at earlier iterations.

Our method provides a vector $\boldsymbol{w}_v$ for each word, which can be regarded as
an embedding of the vth word in the $(M + 1)$-dimensional space. As long as M
is chosen so that the test perplexity is not severely degraded from that of the

---

[3] https://github.com/amueller/word_cloud.

Table 3. The most similar word found by the baseline and our method.

target word	the most similar word	
	baseline	our method
amount	total	total
axis	labels	labels
batch	rscript	rscript
click	button	button
daily	monthly	monthly
height	width	width
predict	models	models
white	black	black
x-axis	y-axis	y-axis

target word	the most similar word	
	baseline	our method
advice	appreciate	suggestion
bottom	position	top
bytes	kb	mb
converting	convert	converted
datetime	posixct	timestamp
environment	calls	global
female	gender	male
integers	integer	non-numeric
json	location	xml
negative	operator	positive
python	array	print
slow	speed	faster
standard	statistics	means

baseline, our method can offer this word embedding as a bonus. Also for the baseline, the vector $\boldsymbol{y}_{.,v} = (y_{1,v}, \ldots, y_{K,v})$ can be regarded as an embedding of the vth word. However, its dimension is equal to K, i.e., the number of latent topics. We checked if the vectors obtained in this manner could be used for finding similar words. In Table 3, the most similar word found by the baseline and our method in terms of Euclidean distance in the embedding space is put on the right hand side of each target word. This result was obtained from the Stack Overflow data set when $K = 128$ and $M = 512$. The baseline and our method sometimes give the same most similar word as shown in the left panel. However, in many cases, the two methods provide different words as shown in the right panel. It should be noted that the dimension M of the embedding achieved by our method can be chosen regardless of K. In contrast, the dimension of the embedding achieved by the baseline is K, i.e., the number of latent topics in LDA. Therefore, it can be said that our method provides an alternative representation of the words away from the latent topics of LDA. Both methods were not so much effective to realize the word-vector arithmetic [12]. It may be required to introduce a mechanism to learn from the word sequence context, which is beyond the scope of this paper.

5   Conclusion

We proposed a new method for estimating the parameters of the per-topic word discrete distributions in LDA by using MLP. The estimation is performed in an online manner by mini-batch gradient ascent. The experimental results showed that there certainly were situations where the proposed method achieved a better test perplexity than the baseline. While the perplexity of CGS could not be improved for many cases, it is an important feature of the baseline and our method to perform the estimation in an online manner. This feature leads to the reduction of the memory consumption.

The improvement when compared to the baseline may be achieved by the factorization $y_{k,v} = \boldsymbol{w}_v \cdot \boldsymbol{t}_k$. This factorization also gives an $(M+1)$-dimensional non-negative vector $\boldsymbol{t}_k$ for each topic in addition to the vector $\boldsymbol{w}_v$. It may also be interesting as a future work to investigate whether this non-negative feature vector obtained for each topic can be used in some text mining applications.

Acknowledgment. This work was supported by JSPS KAKENHI Grant-in-Aid for Scientific Research (C) JP26330256.

References

1. Asuncion, A., Welling, M., Smyth, P., Teh, Y.W.: On smoothing and inference for topic models. In: Proceedings of the Conference on Uncertainty in Artificial Intelligence (UAI), pp. 27–34 (2009)
2. Ba, J.L., Kiros, J.R., Hinton, G.E.: Layer normalization arXiv preprint arXiv:1607.06450 (2016)
3. Blei, D.M., Ng, A.Y., Jordan, M.I.: Latent Dirichlet allocation. J. Mach. Learn. Res. (JMLR) **3**, 993–1022 (2003)
4. Blei, D.M.: Topic modeling and digital humanities. J. Digital Humanit. **2**(1), 8–11 (2013)
5. Duchi, J., Hazan, E., Singer, Y.: Adaptive subgradient methods for online learning and stochastic optimization. J. Mach. Learn. Res. (JMLR) **12**, 2121–2159 (2011)
6. Griffiths, T.L., Steyvers, M.: Finding scientific topics. Proc. National Acad. Sci. (PNAS) **101**(Suppl. 1), 5288–5235 (2004)
7. Grimmer, J., Stewart, B.M.: Text as data: the promise and pitfalls of automatic content analysis methods for political texts. Polit. Anal. **21**(3), 267–297 (2013)
8. Hoffman, M.D., Blei, D.M., Bach, F.: Online learning for latent Dirichlet allocation. In: Proceedings of Neural Information Processing Systems (NIPS), pp. 856–864 (2010)
9. Jacobi, C., van Atteveldt, W., Welbers, K.: Quantitative analysis of large amounts of journalistic texts using topic modelling. Digital Journalism **4**(1), 89–106 (2016)
10. Kingma, D.P., Welling, M.: Auto-encoding variational Bayes. In: Proceedings of the International Conference on Learning Representations (ICLR) (2014)
11. Miao, Y.-S., Yu, L., Blunsom, P.: Neural variational inference for text processing. In: Proceedings of the International Conference on Learning Representations (ICLR) (2016)
12. Mikolov, T., Sutskever, I., Chen, K., Corrado, G.S., Dean, J.: Distributed representations of words and phrases and their compositionality. In: Proceedings of Neural Information Processing Systems (NIPS), pp. 3111–3119 (2013)
13. Nair, V., Hinton, G.E.: Rectified linear units improve restricted Boltzmann machines. In: Proceedings of the 27th International Conference on Machine Learning (ICML), pp. 807–814 (2010)
14. Srivastava, A., Sutton, C.: Neural variational inference for topic models. In: Proceedings of the International Conference on Learning Representations (ICLR) (2017)
15. Srivastava, N., Hinton, G., Krizhevsky, A., Sutskever, I., Salakhutdinov, R.: Dropout: a simple way to prevent neural networks from overfitting. J. Mach. Learn. Res. (JMLR) **15**, 1929–1958 (2014)

GA-Apriori: Combining Apriori Heuristic and Genetic Algorithms for Solving the Frequent Itemsets Mining Problem

Youcef Djenouri[(✉)] and Marco Comuzzi

Ulsan National Institute of Science and Technology (UNIST), 50 UNIST-gil,
Ulju-gun, Ulsan 44949, Republic of Korea
{ydjenouri,mcomuzzi}@unist.ac.kr

Abstract. Finding frequent itemsets is a popular data mining problem, aiming to extract hidden patterns from a transactional database. Several bio-inspired approaches to solve this problem have been proposed to overcome the poor performance of exact algorithms, such as Apriori and FPGrowth. Approaches based on genetic algorithms are among the most efficient ones from the point of view of runtime performance, but they are still inefficient in terms of solution's quality, i.e., the number of frequent itemsets discovered. To deal with this issue, we propose in this paper a new genetic algorithm for finding frequent itemsets called GA-Apriori, in which the crossover and mutation operators are defined by taking into account the Apriori heuristic principle. The results of our evaluation show that GA-Apriori outperforms other approaches to frequent itemset mining based on genetic algorithms, especially when dealing with large instances. The experiments also show that GA-Apriori is competitive with exact approaches in terms of the number of frequent itemsets discovered.

Keywords: Frequent Itemsets Mining · Apriori heuristic · Genetic algorithm

1   Introduction

Frequent Itemsets Mining (FIM) aims to extract frequent itemsets highly correlated from a transactional database. The FIM problem is defined as follows: let T be a set of transactions, $\{T_1, T_2, \ldots, T_m\}$, representing a transactional database, and I be a set of n different items or attributes $\{I_1, I_2, \ldots, I_n\}$. An itemset X is set of items, i.e., $X \subseteq I$. The support of an itemset $X \subseteq I$ is the number of transactions that contain X divided by the number of transactions in T. The itemsets X is called frequent if its support is no less than a user's predefined threshold $MinSup$ [1].

Several FIM algorithms have been proposed. Some of them, such as Apriori [1] and FPGrowth [2], are *exact*, i.e., they generate all frequent itemsets in a database. These algorithms are usually highly time consuming when dealing

© Springer International Publishing AG 2017
U Kang et al. (Eds.): PAKDD 2017 Workshops, LNAI 10526, pp. 138–148, 2017.
DOI: 10.1007/978-3-319-67274-8_13

with large database instances. To overcome this limitation, bio-inspired computational techniques have been applied to FIM, such as genetic and memetic algorithms [3], genetic programming [4,5], or swarm intelligence approaches, e.g., penguin swarm optimization [8], and bee swarm optimization [6,7]. These algorithms perform in reasonable time, but they do not guarantee to find all possible frequent itemsets in a database.

In this paper, we propose a new FIM approach based on genetic algorithms called GA-Apriori. The development of GA-Apriori starts from GA-FIM, that is, a FIM algorithm based on genetic algorithms adapted from Djenouri's et al. [3] genetic algorithm for association rule mining. GA-Apriori extends GA-FIM by taking into account the Apriori heuristic for the definition of the mutation and crossover operators.

GA-Apriori combines the Apriori heuristic with genetic algorithms devising a mining process performed in k steps. For each step i, the *crossover* operator allows to generate the itemsets of size i from the frequent itemsets of size $(i-1)$, while the *mutation* operator allows to find frequent itemsets from the itemsets generated by the crossover operator.

To validate the performance and the quality of the suggested approach, intensive experiments have been run on real data instances. The results show that GA-Apriori outperforms GA-FIM in terms of the number of frequent itemsets discovered. Moreover, it outperforms Apriori and FPGrowth algorithms in terms of computational time. The results also reveal that GA-Apriori is competitive compared to exact approaches, such as Apriori and FPGrowth, in respect of the quality of solution, i.e., the number of frequent itemsets discovered.

The remainder of the paper is organized as follows: Sect. 2 reviews the existing genetic approaches for solving the FIM problem. Sections 3 and 4 describe respectively GA-FIM and the Apriori heuristic. GA-Apriori is presented in Sect. 5. The performance evaluation is provided in Sect. 6, and finally, Sect. 7 draws the conclusions.

2 Related Work

Solutions to the FIM problem can be divided into two categories, i.e., exact and bio-inspired. Exact approaches aim to extract all frequent itemsets in a database. Example of exact approaches are Apriori [1] and FPgrowth [2]. These algorithms are highly time and memory consuming.

Bio-inspired approaches utilize computational techniques inspired by nature, such as swarm intelligence (BSO [6], HBSO-TS [7], PeSOA [8]) or evolutionary approaches (GAR [9] and GENAR [10]) to solve the FIM problem. Since this paper focuses on applications of genetic algorithms to the FIM problem, in the remainder of this section we concentrate on existing genetic algorithm-based approaches to FIM.

The first two genetic algorithms for FIM proposed in the literature are GENAR [10] and GAR [9]. Their main limit is the inefficient representation of the individual solution. In [11], the authors propose an algorithm based on genetic algorithm called ARMGA. In [12], AGA, also based on genetic algorithms, is developed for computing FIM. The two major differences between classical ARMGA and AGA are the mutation and crossover operators. The algorithm PQGMA is proposed by Liu for FIM in [13]. Mainly, the mining process is performed by applying classical GA, while the mutation and the crossover operations use simulated annealing and computing strategy principals, respectively. However, the use of quantum computing in the mutation suffers from diversification and therefore leads to premature convergence.

The approach proposed by [16] uses an adaptive mutation rate, which provides an important population variation. Nevertheless, the mutation probability is computed at each iteration, thus increasing the computational time.

Romero et al. developed G3PARM based on genetic programming [15]. They use the G3P (Grammar Guided Genetic Programming) to avoid generating invalid individuals. Also G3PARM permits multiple variants of data by using a context free grammar.

An interesting work providing a performance analysis of generic algorithm-based approaches to FIM is [14]. The results reveal that GA-based algorithms outperform the exact methods in terms of computational time. Nevertheless, GA-based algorithms return only a limited number of frequent itemsets. This can be explained by the fact that these algorithms explore the solutions space of the itemsets using randomness and often ignoring the intrinsic properties of the FIM problem. To deal with this issue, we propose in this paper, an improved genetic algorithm for FIM problem that uses the Apriori heuristic in the generation process. Before presenting our contribution, in the next two sections, we briefly present the preliminaries of our work, that is, GA-FIM and the Apriori heuristic.

3   GA-FIM: Genetic Algorithm for FIM

In [3], the authors have proposed IARMGA, that is, a genetic algorithm-based approach to solve the association rule mining problem. GA-FIM, which we extend in this paper, is a straightforward adaptation of IARMGA to the FIM problem. The remainder of this section briefly describes the GA-FIM algorithm.

The aim of GA-FIM is to find in a reasonable time one part of the frequent itemsets in a database respecting the minimum support constraint. The initial population of *PopSize* itemsets is first randomly generated considering each itemset as a vector of n elements. The ith element is set to 1 if the ith item belongs to an itemset, and to 0 otherwise. The crossover and the mutation operators are then applied. The crossover combines two itemsets in order to produce two other itemsets (intensification), while the mutation operator flips one bit of each generated itemset (diversification).

More in detail, the main operators of GA-FIM are defined as follows:

1. **Crossover:** The classical crossover is applied for each two itemsets selected from the population. For instance if the parent itemsets are $t_1 = \{0, 1, 0, 1, 1\}$

and $t_2 = \{1, 0, 0, 0, 1\}$, and the crossover point is 3, then two other itemsets are generated, which are $t_3 = \{0, 1, 0, 0, 1\}$ and $t_4 = \{1, 0, 0, 1, 1\}$.

2. **Mutation:** Similar to the crossover, the mutation is applied on each generated itemsets, as in the classical genetic algorithm. For instance, if we have the two itemsets generated previously by the crossover operator, and the mutation point is also 3, then, two new itemsets are produced: $t_5 = \{0, 1, 1, 0, 1\}$ and $t_6 = \{1, 0, 1, 1, 1\}$.

At the end of each iteration, the selection operation is performed to keep only *PopSize* itemsets for the next iteration. The selection is executed using the support of the given itemset as fitness function. This process (crossover, mutation, selection) is repeated for a fixed maximum number of iterations. The set of all frequent itemsets is the union of all frequents itemsets found.

4   Apriori Heuristic

The Apriori algorithm [1] is a well known exact FIM approach that finds all frequent itemsets in a transactional database that satisfy a minimum support user's threshold *MinSup*. The goal of the Apriori heuristic is to reduce the search space to find frequent itemsets by exploring recursively the candidate itemsets. The principle is that an itemset of size k is frequent if and only if all its subsets are frequents. Thus, at each iteration k, the candidates itemsets of size k are generated by joining two frequent itemsets of size $k - 1$. This process should be repeated until the candidate itemsets of length k is empty.

Let us consider the following example containing 5 transactions $\{T_1:\{a, b\}, T_2:\{b, c, d\}, T_3:\{a, b, c\}, T_4:\{e\}, T_5:\{c, d, e\}\}$.

Figure 1 illustrates the results of Apriori using the set of transactions described above and with minimum support equal to 40%. The transactional database is first scanned to calculate the support of each candidate itemset of

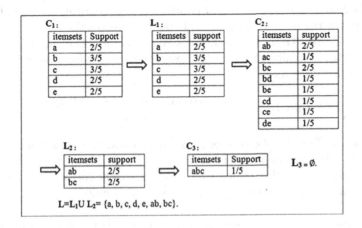

Fig. 1. Apriori heuristic illustration

size 1 (candidate itemset containing only one item). The frequent itemsets of size 1 are then extracted. In this example, all candidates itemsets are frequent because their supports are greater than 0.4. In the second iteration, the candidate itemsets of size 2 are extracted by joining the frequent itemsets of size 1. The support of each candidates itemsets of size 2 is computed and then extract the frequent itemsets of size 2, these two frequent itemsets are $\{ab, bc, cd\}$. We join these two frequent itemsets obtaining the candidate itemsets $\{abc, abd, bcd\}$. The support of these itemsets is less than 0.4, i.e., no new itemset is frequent, so the process is stopped. The set of all frequent itemsets is the union of the frequent itemsets of size 1 and size 2, that is, $\{a, b, c, d, e, ab, bc, cd\}$.

5   GA-Apriori: A Genetic FIM Approach Using the Apriori Heuristic

The proposed GA-Apriori approach uses the Apriori heuristic to improve the itemsets space exploration in GA-FIM. The aim is to use the Apriori heuristic in designing the genetic algorithm operators for exploring only the frequent itemsets. GA-Apriori adopts the overall process typical of FIM approaches inspired by genetic algorithms. However, GA-Apriori's operator differs from the classical genetic algorithm in the way that the initialization, fitness computing, crossover, mutation, and selection operators are defined. These are described in detail in the following.

1. **Population Initialization.** The initial population is determined by choosing *PopSize* frequent items. To do so, the frequent itemsets of size 1 are computed and sorted according to the support constraint. Then, the first *PopSize* frequent items are kept, the other frequent items are removed. For instance, let us consider 5 items $\{a, b, c, d, e\}$ with the following supports $\{sup(a) = 0.5, sup(b) = 0.3, sup(c) = 0.6, sup(d) = 0.8, sup(e) = 0.2\}$. With $MinSup = 0.4$, the following frequent items are determined: $\{a, c, d\}$, now if the $PopSize = 2$ then, the initial population is constituted by $(0, 0, 0, 1, 0)$ to represent the item d and $(0, 0, 1, 0, 0)$ to represent the item c.

2. **Fitness Computing.** The fitness of a given itemset t is equal to its support if it reaches the minimum support constraint, otherwise it is equal to -1. More formally, we have:

$$Fitness(t) = \begin{cases} support(t) & \text{if } support(t) \geq MinSup; \\ -1 & \text{Otherwise.} \end{cases}$$

3. **Crossover.** The aim of crossover is to generate two candidate itemsets of size k from two frequent itemsets of size $(k-1)$. Two parents are first selected from a given population, then, to create new children, the following two crossover constraints inspired by the Apriori heuristic are applied:

   - All items of the first parent are copied to the first children, and all items of the second parent are copied to the second children.

– Choose one item e_1 equal to 1 in the second parent which evaluates to 0 in the first parent and modify the value of e_1 in the first child to 1. Similarly, choose one item e_2 equal to 1 in the first parent and to 0 in the second parent and modify the value of e_2 in the second child by one.

For instance, let us consider 5 items $\{a, b, c, d, e\}$ and the two parents $Parent_1 = \{0, 0, 0, 1, 0\}$, representing the itemset (ab), and $Parent_2 = \{0, 0, 1, 0, 0\}$, representing the itemset (cd). If we choose $e_1 = c$ and $e_2 = b$ then, the two children $child_1$ and $child_2$ are generated as $child_1 = \{1, 1, 1, 0, 0\}$, representing the itemset (abc), and $child_2 = \{0, 1, 1, 1, 0\}$, representing the itemset (bcd).

4. **Mutation.** The aim of mutation is to generate frequent itemsets of size k from infrequent itemsets of the same size. For each generated itemset obtained applying the crossover operator, if an infrequent itemset $indiv$ of size k is found, then, two items e_1 equal to 1 and e_2 equal to 0 in $indiv$ are chosen. The values of the chosen items is flipped, that is, item e_1 is set to 0 and e_2 is set to 1 in $indiv$. This operation is repeated until an itemset of size k is found.

   For instance, let us consider 5 items $\{a, b, c, d, e\}$ and the itemset $indiv = \{0, 0, 1, 1, 1\}$, representing the itemset (cde). If we choose $e_1 = c$ and $e_2 = a$ then, $indiv = \{1, 0, 0, 1, 1\}$, which represents the itemset (ade). If this itemset is frequent, then the process is stopped. Otherwise, the process is repeated until a frequent itemset of size 3 is found.

5. **Selection.** The selection operator aims to select the best frequent itemsets generated by the crossover and the mutation operators. Indeed, the best $PopSize$ frequent itemsets are kept to be the new population of the next iteration.

The GA-Apriori algorithm is shown in Algorithm 1.

GA-Apriori requires as input a transactional database T for computing the support of the generated itemsets, and the minimum support value $MinSup$ to determine the frequent itemsets. It also requires two internal vectors $CurrentPopulation$ and $NewPopulation$ to store the current population and new population with their cost (i.e., their support). The algorithm returns the set of all frequent itemsets F.

First, the frequent items of size 1 are determined using the function FindFrequentOneItemset(), which enumerates all items and then computes the support of each item, extracting the frequent items. It then sorts the frequent items according to their support. The first $PopSize$ frequent items are assigned to the $CuurentPopulation$. The latter is added to the set of frequent itemsets F.

Afterwards, the crossover operation is applied on each pair of parents in the current population. The result of the crossover is added to the new population $NewPopulation$.

The next step is to refine the new population using the mutation operator by transforming the infrequent itemsets into frequent itemsets. The new population $NewPopulation$ modified by the mutation operator is added to the set of frequent itemsets F. $NewPopulation$ becomes the current population for the next iteration using the selection procedure. The overall process is repeated until the $CurrentPopulation$ vector is empty.

Algorithm 1. GA-Apriori Algorithm

1: **Input**: T: Transactional database. MinSup: Minimum Support user's threshold.
2: **Output** :F: The set of frequent Itemsets.
3: $F \leftarrow \emptyset$.
4: CurrentPopulation $\leftarrow$ FindFrequentOneItemset().
5: **while** CurrentPopulation $\not\in \emptyset$ **do**
6:    $F \leftarrow F \cup$ CurrentPopulation.
7:    NewPopulation $\leftarrow \emptyset$.
8:    **for** each two individual $(parent_1, parent_2) \in$ CurrentPopulation **do**
9:       NewPopulation $\leftarrow$ NewPopulation $\cup$ Crossover($Parent_1, Parent_2$).
10:    **end for**
11:    **for** each infrequent $indiv \in NewPopulation$ **do**
12:       **while** infrequent $indiv$ **do**
13:          Mutation($indiv$)
14:       **end while**
15:    **end for**
16:    $F \leftarrow F \cup$ NewPopulation.
17:    CurrentPopulation $\leftarrow$ Selection(NewPopulation).
18: **end while**
19: **return** F

---

6   Experimental Results

To validate GA-Apriori, intensive experiments have been carried out. Algorithms have been implemented in C++ and experiments run on a desktop machine equipped with Intel $I3$ processor and 4 GB memory. First, some experiments have been run to tune the population's size of GA-Apriori. Then, the performance of GA-Apriori is compared to GAFIM and other exact approaches, i.e., Apriori and FPGrowth, using real scientific databases frequently used for benchmarking FIM research [17].

6.1   Parameter Setting for GA-Apriori

To set the population's size, we have run a benchmark experiment using the IBM-Quest database. Specifically, the population's size is chosen by considering the average support of the frequent itemsets discovered in respect of the runtime required to discover frequent itemsets.

Figures 2 and 3 present, respectively, the average support of the frequent itemsets and the runtime in seconds of the GA-Apriori approach using the IBM-Quest instance containing 1000 transactions and 40 different items. By varying the population's size from 10 to 100, the average support saturates at 40 individuals, whereas the runtime increases by enhancing the population's size. Consequently, the population's size of GA-Apriori is set to 40 for the remainder of the experimental evaluation.

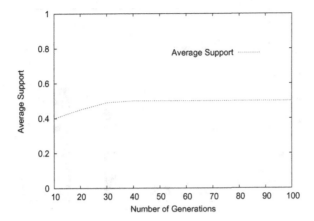

Fig. 2. The average supports of frequent itemsets found by GA-Apriori for different number of iterations using IBM-Quest instance

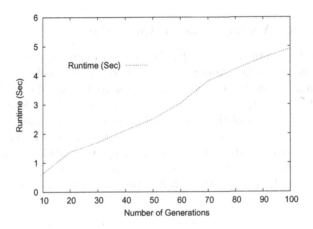

Fig. 3. Runtime (Sec) of GA-Apriori approach for different number of iterations using IBM-Quest instance

6.2   Performance Analysis: GA-Apriori vs GA-FIM

Figures 4 shows the number of frequent itemsets found by GA-Apriori and GA-FIM approaches for different instances. The population size of both approaches is set to 40, and the minimum support is set to 10%. According to this figure, we remark that GA-Apriori outperforms GA-FIM in terms of frequent itemsets found for all instances used. Indeed, the number of frequent itemsets of GA-Apriori exceeds 22000 when using the instance IBM-Artificial containing 100000 transactions and 999 items. However, the number of frequent itemsets of GA-FIM does not reach 15000. These results are obtained thanks to the Apriori heuristic used in the searching of frequent itemsets by the genetic algorithm in GA-Apriori.

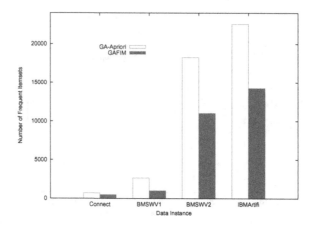

Fig. 4. The number of frequent itemsets found by GA-Apriori and GAFIM approaches for different used instances

6.3 GA-Apriori VS Exact-Based Approaches

Figures 5 and 6 present, respectively, the number of frequent itemsets and the runtime in seconds of GA-Apriori compared to Apriori and FPGrowth using different instances. The minimum support is set to 40% in all experiments. The results show that GA-Apriori converges to the optimal solution found by Apriori and FPGrowth in terms of the number of frequent itemsets found. Indeed, the difference between our approach and the exact approaches does not exceed 100 frequent itemsets in all data instances used, except the IBM-Artificial, for which the difference is 116 frequent itemsets. The results also reveal that, as expected, GA-Apriori outperforms the exact approaches in terms of computational time.

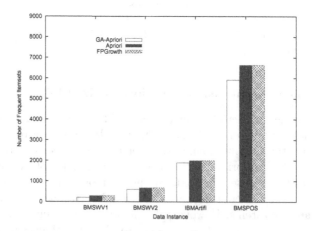

Fig. 5. The number of frequent itemsets found by GA-Apriori and exact-based approaches for different used instances

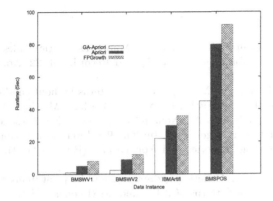

Fig. 6. Runtime (Sec) of GA-Apriori and exact-based approaches for different used instances

For the BMS-POS instance (which includes more than 500000 transactions and more than 1600 items), the runtime of FPGrowth is twice more than GA-Apriori. These results are reached thanks again to the efficient heuristic applied in the search process combined with the use of genetic algorithm to find frequent itemsets.

7 Conclusions

In this paper, a new genetic algorithm approach called GA-Apriori for the frequent itemset mining problem is proposed. The solutions space is explored intelligently by combining Apriori heuristic and genetic algorithms. The mining process is performed in k steps; for each step i the crossover operator allows to generate the itemsets of size i from the frequent itemsets of size $(i-1)$, while the mutation operator allows to find frequent itemsets from the itemsets generated by the crossover operator.

To analyze the behavior of the proposed approach, several experiments have been carried out on real data instances. The results show that GA-Apriori outperforms GA-FIM in terms of the number of frequent itemsets. Moreover, it outperforms the exact approaches Apriori and FPGrowth in terms of computational time. The results also reveal that GA-Apriori is competitive compared to the exact approaches for the quality of the solutions found.

As future work, we plan to employ the Apriori heuristic in other bio-inspired approaches, such as swarm intelligence algorithms and test our approach for solving big domain-specific complex problems, such as those related to business intelligence and mining of information systems event logs for process mining.

References

1. Agrawal, R., Imielinski, T., Swami, A.: Mining association rules between sets of items in large databases. In: ACM Sigmod Record, vol. 22, No. 2, pp. 207–216. ACM, June 1993
2. Han, J., Pei, J., Yin, Y.: Mining frequent patterns without candidate generation. In: ACM Sigmod Record, vol. 29, No. 2, pp. 1–12. ACM, May 2000
3. Djenouri, Y., Bendjoudi, A., Nouali-Taboudjemat, N.: Association rules mining using evolutionary algorithms. In: The 9th International Conference on Bio-inspired Computing: Theories and Applications (BIC-TA 2014). LNCS, October 2014
4. Smart, O., Burrell, L.: Genetic programming and frequent itemset mining to identify feature selection patterns of iEEG and fMRI epilepsy data. Eng. Appl. Artif. Intell. **39**, 198–214 (2015)
5. Luna, J.M., Pechenizkiy, M., Ventura, S.: Mining exceptional relationships with grammar-guided genetic programming. Knowl. Inf. Syst. **47**(3), 571–594 (2016)
6. Djenouri, Y., Drias, H., Habbas, Z.: Bees swarm optimisation using multiple strategies for association rule mining. Int. J. Bio-Inspired Comput. **6**(4), 239–249 (2014)
7. Djenouri, Y., Drias, H., Habbas, Z.: Hybrid intelligent method for association rules mining using multiple strategies. Int. J. Appl. Metaheuristic Comput. (IJAMC) **5**(1), 46–64 (2014)
8. Gheraibia, Y., Moussaoui, A., Djenouri, Y., Kabir, S., Yin, P.Y.: Penguins search optimisation algorithm for association rules mining. CIT. J. Comput. Inform. Technol. **24**(2), 165–179 (2016)
9. Mata J., Alvarez J., and Riquelme J.: An Evolutionary algorithm to discover numeric association rules. In: Proceedings of the ACM Symposium on Applied Computing SAC, pp. 590–594 (2002)
10. Mata, J., Alvarez, J., Riquelme, J.: Mining numeric association rules with genetic algorithms. In: Proceedings of the International Conference ICANNGA, pp. 264–267 (2001)
11. Yan, X., Zhang, C.: Genetic algorithm based strategy for identifying association rule without specifying minimum support. Expert Syst. Appl. **36**(2), 3066–3076 (2009)
12. wang, M., zou, Q., Lin, C.: Multi dimensions association rules mining on adaptive genetic algorithm. In: International Conference on Uncertainly Reasoning on Knowledge Engineering IEEE (2011)
13. Liu, D.: Improved genetic algorithm based on simulated annealing and quantum computing strategy for association rule mining. J. Softw. **5**(11), 1243–1249 (2010)
14. Indira, K., Kanmani, S.: Performance analysis of genetic algorithm for mining association rules. Int. J. Comput. Sci. Issues **9**(1) (2012)
15. Romero, C., Zafra, A., Luna, J., Ventura, S.: Association rule mining using genetic programming to provide feedback to instructors from multiple-choice quiz data. J. Expert Syst. **30**, 162–172 (2012)
16. Hong, G., Zhou, Y.: An algorithm for mining association rules based on improved genetic algorithm and its application. In: Third International Conference on Genetic and Evolutionary Computing, pp. 117–120. IEEE Computer Science (2009)
17. Guvenir, H.A., Uysal, I.: Bilkent university function approximation repository. 20120312 (2000). http://funapp.CS.bilkent.edu.tr/DataSets

DM-BPM

Shelf Time Analysis in CTP Insurance Claims Processing

Robert Andrews[✉] and Moe Wynn

Queensland University of Technology, Brisbane, QLD 4000, Australia
{r.andrews,m.wynn}@qut.edu.au

Abstract. Shelf time (idle time that exceeds acceptable duration) can contribute (significantly) to overall process execution time. In this paper we describe a process mining-based approach to shelf time analysis. The technique takes as input an *event log* extracted from historical executions of a business process and requires each event have timestamp attributes representing both the start and completion times of each event. The essence of our shelf time identification technique is finding events which do not temporally overlap other events in the same case in the log. The major contributions of this paper include (i) an approach for identifying and quantifying periods of shelf time in an event log triggered by an event activity, (ii) an analysis of a portfolio of claims of commercial CTP insurer to identify shelf time periods and triggering activities and (iii) a discussion of an extension of the approach to include identification of shelf time periods associated with other event attributes, e.g. the resource. The technique was applied to a real life log extracted from a Queensland CTP insurer and was able to identify activities that triggered shelf time periods and to quantify the pervasiveness of shelf time across activities and cases in the log.

Keywords: Process mining · Shelf time analysis

1 Introduction

A business process is an inter-related set of steps designed to transform inputs into outputs (goods or services). Understanding how a processes works (process analysis) is a key step in determining how the process can be improved (i.e. be changed so that it works somehow 'better'). Process analysis then involves identifying performance metrics that allow point-in-time monitoring and tracking over time to assess how well a business process is meetings its proposed objectives. Such metrics may include various times associated with process execution, e.g. throughput time or idle time.

Shelf time is any idle-time period i.e. *no activity* is recorded on a case, where the duration of the idle-time exceeds some process-specific threshold and becomes somehow unacceptable (to process stakeholders). Clearly, periods of shelf time will (usually negatively) impact on individual case durations. While potentially significant at an individual case level, it is also important to be able

© Springer International Publishing AG 2017
U Kang et al. (Eds.): PAKDD 2017 Workshops, LNAI 10526, pp. 151–162, 2017.
DOI: 10.1007/978-3-319-67274-8_14

to determine the prevalence and impact of shelf time across the entire corpus of process cases. Our shelf time analysis method focuses on identifying delays following the *completion* of activities and thus is useful in revealing activities that are responsible for *causing* process instance delays. We argue that the identification of such activities is important as they represent break points in a process instance beyond which it is not possible or practical to continue until some 'blocking factor' is resolved. We note that the existence of shelf time periods may be an indicator that a process is *resource bound* i.e. not enough capacity to deal with an accumulation of cases completing to the point where a shelf time period is observed, or that there is some *external or un-recorded* (in the event log) activity which is occurring, and on which the process depends. Consider, for instance, an insurance claims officer requesting a report from an independent medical examiner regarding the extent of the claimant's injuries before determining a compensation offer. From the claims officer's point of view, the (external) procedure at the medical examiner's practice is opaque and the claims officer cannot proceed with the claim until the report is received. There is then shelf time, i.e. a break in the process, associated with the activity of requesting a report from the medical examiner.

An understanding of the root causes of shelf time periods provides insights useful to process stakeholders and analysts as input to process improvement/re-design. Questions that may be of interest in attempting to derive the root causes of shelf time periods include (i) are there activities frequently associated with shelf time periods? (ii) are cases with significant shelf time periods associated with particular resources? (iii) are interactions with particular third parties associated with shelf time periods?

In this paper we take a process-mining based approach to identifying and quantifying the effects of shelf time on case duration. The major contributions of this paper include (i) an approach for identifying and quantifying periods of shelf time in an event log triggered by an event activity, (ii) an analysis of a portfolio of claims of commercial CTP insurer to identify shelf time periods and triggering activities and (iii) a discussion of an extension of the approach to include identification of shelf time periods associated with other event attributes, e.g. the resource.

The remainder of this paper is organised as follows. In Sect. 2 we discuss some previous work related to idle-time analysis. In Sect. 3 we define the elements of our approach including events, event log, activities and resources and outline our algorithm for detecting shelf time periods (and associated triggering activities) in any case. In Sect. 4 we provide results from the application of our approach to real-life logs provided by a commercial CTP insurer and in Sect. 5 we reflect on the case study and provide some direction for future work in this area.

2   Related Work

Operations management is primarily concerned with efficiently controlling business processes in the production of goods or the delivery of services (the focus of the particular process). Its goal is the efficient use of resources in meeting customer requirements. In Operations Management, *idle time* is defined as *(cycle time - processing time)* where *cycle time* is the time between output of two *flow units* (outputs of the process, e.g. products or delivered services) and *processing time* is the actual time spent in each of the activities making up the process.

Idle time has long been of interest in process analysis in a variety of industries. In [2], the authors used simulation models to derive a set of variables useful in reducing doctor's idle time in an outpatient setting. In [11] the authors use image processing-based methodology to automatically quantify the idle time of hydraulic excavators and in [5] the authors anlayse cycle time and idle time of draglines with a view to increasing efficient use of such capital intensive equipment.

Process mining, a branch of data science, aims at utilising historical, process-related information captured in so-called *event logs* to discover, monitor and improve processes [1]. Process mining is becoming more popular as evidenced by the growing number of case studies detailing successful application of analysis techniques [3,4,9,10]. Process mining however, in common with other forms of data analysis, as is pointed out in [7,8], is hampered by the overall data quality of the event log and the limited information frequently found in event logs, particularly those not generated by process-aware information systems. In [8] the authors refer to the common problem of not having exhaustive timestamp information recorded for events (i.e. having only a completed timestamp rather than scheduled, started and completed times).

In [6] the authors investigate the applicability of process mining approach to the semi-structured test processes of ASML (the leading manufacturer of wafer scanners in the world) with the aim of analysing idle time. Here the authors modify the original event log by applying an 'inversion filter' to the activities in the log such that revised activities represent the transition from one activity in a case to the next activity allowing the analysis of idle times instead of activity durations.

3   Formalisations

Definition 1 (Attribute, Event, Event Log). Let $\mathscr{E}$ be the *event universe*, i.e. the set of all possible event identifiers. Events may be characterised by various *attributes*, e.g. an event may belong to a particular case, have a timestamp, correspond to an activity, and can be executed by a particular person.

Let $AN = \{a_1, a_2, ..., a_n\}$ be a set of all possible attribute names. For each attribute $a_i \in AN$ ($1 \leq i \leq n$), $\mathcal{D}_{a_i}$ is its domain, i.e. the set of all possible values for the attribute a_i.

For any event $e \in \mathscr{E}$ and an attribute name $a \in AN$: $\#_a(e) \in \mathcal{D}_a$ is the value of attribute named a for event e. If an event e does not have an attribute named a, then $\#_a(e) = \bot$ (null value).

Let $\mathcal{D}_{id}$ be the set of event identifiers, $\mathcal{D}_{case}$ be the set of case identifiers, $\mathcal{D}_{act}$ be the set of activity names, and $\mathcal{D}_{time}$ be the set of possible timestamps,

$\mathcal{D}_{res}$ be the set of resource identifiers. For each event $e \in \mathcal{E}$, we define a number of standard attributes:

- $\#_{id}(e) \in \mathcal{D}_{id}$ is the event identifier of e;
- $\#_{case}(e) \in \mathcal{D}_{case}$ is the case identifier of e;
- $\#_{act}(e) \in \mathcal{D}_{act}$ is the activity name of e;
- $\#_{start}(e) \in \mathcal{D}_{time}$ is the starting time of e;
- $\#_{complete}(e) \in \mathcal{D}_{time}$ is the completion time of e; and
- $\#_{res}(e) \in \mathcal{D}_{res}$ is the resource who triggered the occurrence of e.

An event log $\mathcal{L} \subseteq \mathcal{E}$ is a set of events. This definition of an event log allows the log to be viewed as a table, thus allowing the application of relational algebra to the log.

Definition 2 (Shelf Time Period). Let $\mathcal{L} \subseteq \mathcal{E}$ be an event log, $AN_{\mathcal{L}}$ be a set of attribute names found in $\mathcal{L}$ and $\mathcal{D}_a$ be the set of all possible values of $a \in AN_{\mathcal{L}}$. Let $\mathcal{D}_{case}$ be the set of all case values in $\mathcal{L}$ and $\mathcal{D}_{time}$ be the set of possible event timestamps in log $\mathcal{L}$. Let θ be the duration of a time window and $\delta(t_1, t_2)$ give the difference between two times, t_1 and t_2, where $t_1 \leq t_2$.

A *shelf time period* is present in log $\mathcal{L}$ if:

- $\exists e_i, e_j \in \mathcal{L} | \neg \exists e_n \in \mathcal{L}, (\#_{id}(e_i) \neq \#_{id}(e_j) \neq \#_{id}(e_n)) \wedge (\#_{case}(e_i) = \#_{case}(e_j) = \#_{case}(e_n)) \wedge (\#_{complete}(e_n) > \#_{complete}(e_i)) \wedge (\#_{start}(e_n) < \#_{start}(e_j)) \wedge \delta(\#_{complete}(e_i), \#_{start}(e_j)) > \theta$

That is, a shelf time period is present in a log, if there exists events e_i and e_j such that there does not exist any other event e_n where e_i, e_j and e_n are in the same case, and that e_n is never concurrent with either e_i or e_j and the time difference between the completion of e_i and the start of e_j exceeds some process-dependent value, θ. **Note** that if θ is very small, then shelf time is the same as idle time.

Shelf time periods in the log may occur in a number of scenarios as shown in Fig. 1. In the illustration, the solid bars represent activities in a single case with (i) the length of the bar representing the duration of the activity, (ii) the horizontal alignment of the bars representing the relative timing of each activity in the case. This means that bars that align vertically on their left edges have a simultaneous start time, while bars that align vertically on their right edges have a simultaneous complete time. Shelf time periods may be bounded by the completion of a single event (marking the beginning of a shelf time period) and the start of a single event (marking the end of the shelf time period) as illustrated in scenario 1. Alternate scenarios allow for shelf time periods to begin with multiple events completing simultaneously or end with multiple events beginning simultaneously as shown in scenarios 2, 3 and 4.

Definition 3 (Shelf Time Period Associated With a Given Activity). It is possible to filter shelf time periods to those that are triggered by the completion of a given activity.

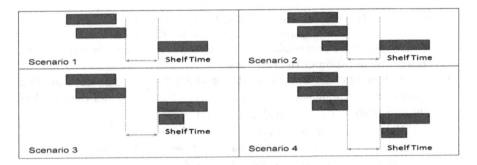

Fig. 1. Shelf time scenarios

Let $\mathcal{L} \subseteq \mathcal{E}$ be an event log, $AN_{\mathcal{L}}$ be a set of attribute names found in $\mathcal{L}$ and $\mathcal{D}_a$ be the set of all possible values of $a \in AN_{\mathcal{L}}$. Let $\mathcal{D}_{case}$ be the set of all case values in $\mathcal{L}$, $\mathcal{D}_{act}$ be the set of all activities in $\mathcal{L}$ and $\mathcal{D}_{time}$ be the set of possible event timestamps in log $\mathcal{L}$.

A *shelf time period*, triggered by a particular activity $act_x \in \mathcal{D}_{act}$ is present in log $\mathcal{L}$ if:

– $\exists e_i, e_j \in \mathcal{L}, \#_{act}(e_i) = act_x | \neg \exists e_n \in \mathcal{L}, (\#_{id}(e_i) \neq \#_{id}(e_j) \neq \#_{id}(e_n)) \wedge$
$(\#_{case}(e_i) = \#_{case}(e_j) = \#_{case}(e_n)) \wedge (\#_{complete}(e_n) > \#_{complete}(e_i)) \wedge$
$(\#_{start}(e_n) < \#_{start}(e_j)) \wedge \delta(\#_{complete}(e_i), \#_{start}(e_j)) > \theta$

Definition 4 (Shelf Time Period Associated With A Given Resource).
It is possible to identify shelf time periods associated with a given resource. Here we consider that a resource may be assigned to a portfolio of *concurrently active* cases.

Let $\mathcal{L} \subseteq \mathcal{E}$ be an event log, $AN_{\mathcal{L}}$ be a set of attribute names found in $\mathcal{L}$ and $\mathcal{D}_a$ be the set of all possible values of $a \in AN_{\mathcal{L}}$. Let $\mathcal{D}_{res}$ be the set of all resource identifiers in $\mathcal{L}$ and $\mathcal{D}_{time}$ be the set of possible event start timestamps in log $\mathcal{L}$.

A *shelf time period*, associated with a particular resource $res_i \in \mathcal{D}_{res}$ is present in log $\mathcal{L}$ if:

– $\exists e_i, e_j \in \mathcal{L}, \#_{res}(e_i) = \#_{res}(e_j) = res_x | \neg \exists e_n \in \mathcal{L}, (\#_{id}(e_i) \neq \#_{id}(e_j) \neq$
$\#_{id}(e_n)) \wedge (\#_{complete}(e_n) > \#_{complete}(e_i)) \wedge (\#_{start}(e_n) < \#_{start}(e_j)) \wedge$
$\delta(\#_{complete}(e_i), \#_{start}(e_j)) > \theta$

3.1 Approach

Periods of shelf time associated with activities may be identified and the pervasiveness of shelf time in the event log may be determined using the following three step approach:

1. Populate a table, ST, containing events that are shelf time 'triggers', i.e. events that do not temporally overlap other events in the same case

- $ST \equiv \mathcal{L} - \Pi_{a.*}(\sigma_{a.case=b.case \wedge a.id \neq b.id \wedge b.start \leq a.complete}$
$$\wedge b.complete > a.complete(\rho_a(\mathcal{L}) \times \rho_b(\mathcal{L})))$$

2. For each event in ST, determine the temporally 'next' event in the case and determine the duration of the shelf time.

(a) For each event $e_i \in ST$, build a table of all events e_j, in the same case, that start after e_i completes, i.e. $\#_{complete}(e_i) < \#_{start}(e_j)$, and the calculate the difference $\delta(\#_{complete}(e_i), \#_{start}(e_j))$

- $BA \equiv \Pi_{ST.id,ST.case,ST.act,\mathcal{L}.id,\mathcal{L}.act,\delta(ST.complete,\mathcal{L}.start)}$
$$(\sigma_{ST.case=\mathcal{L}.case \wedge \mathcal{L}.start > ST.complete}(ST \times \mathcal{L}))$$

- $\rho_{ST.id/startid,ST.case/case,ST.act/startact,\mathcal{L}.id/nextid,\mathcal{L}.act/nextact,}$
$$\delta(ST.complete,\mathcal{L}.start)/shelftime(BA)$$

(b) For each $startid$ in BA, find the $nextid$ with the minimum $shelftime$, i.e. the temporally next event. Populate a table, $ActivityShelf$, with only these events.

- $ActivityShelf \equiv \Pi_{case,startact,nextact,shelftime}(BA)-$
$\Pi_{x.case,x.startact,x.nextact,x.shelftime}$
$$(\sigma_{x.case=y.case \wedge x.startact=y.startact \wedge x.shelftime > y.shelftime}$$
$$(\rho_x(BA) \times \rho_y(BA)))$$

3. Aggregate $ActivityShelf$ as required.

4   Case Study

The Compulsory Third Party (CTP) scheme operating in Queensland (Australia) provides motor vehicle owners and drivers an unlimited liability policy for personal injury caused through the use of the insured vehicle in incidents to which the governing legislation, the Motor Accident Insurance Act 1994 (the Act) applies. The Queensland CTP scheme is managed by the Motor Accident Insurance Commission (MAIC) and is underwritten by (currently four) licensed, commercial insurers. CTP premiums, collected as a component of vehicle registration, contribute to the respective insurers premium pool and are used to pay compensation to accident victims.

The Act lays out in detail the rights and obligations of the parties involved (claimant and insurer) in lodging and settling a compensation claim for injuries received as a result of a motor vehicle accident. The claimant must first **notify** the relevant insurer of their intention seek compensation (by lodging a standard Notification of Accident Claim form). The insurer will assess the claim to determine that it **complies** with the provisions of the Act. The insurer will then make determination as to whether it is **liable** for the claim, i.e. the insurer has accepted the application for insurance from the claimant. Following the liability decision, the claimant and the insurer will **negotiate** the agreed compensation (usually at a conference but negotiation may include litigation if the parties cannot come to agreement). Once agreed, formal **settlement** of the claim takes place and, after all monies are disbursed, the claim is **finalised**. A claim may exit the process at each of the Notification, Compliance and Liability phases. Reasons for exiting the claim process include the claim failing to comply with the provisions of the Act (through not containing all information relevant to the claim or not being submitted within prescribed timeframes) or the nominated insurer determining it is not liable for the claim (through the 'at fault' driver not holding a valid, current CTP insurance policy with the nominated insurer).

Once the insurer has accepted liability, the claim will progress to completion. Figure 2 shows the phased nature of the CTP claims management process.

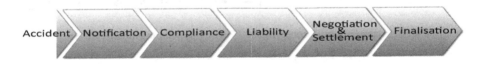

Fig. 2. CTP claims management - value chain

For any of the scheme insurers, the injury-compensation claims process is complex involving negotiations between multiple parties (e.g. claimants, other insurers, law firms, health services providers, Centrelink, Workers Compensation, hospitals, police). While the Act prescribes maximum allowed periods for claims to reach certain milestones, CTP insurers nevertheless experience significant behavioural and performance variations in CTP claims processing affecting, in particular, claim durations. For instance, of the 2,535 settled claims in the dataset used for this study where the maximum injury severity was rated minimal, the duration from notification to settlement ranged from a minimum of 0 months to a maximum of 131 months (median duration = 19 months, mean duration = 21 months).

The CTP injury compensation claims process may be considered as a phased process marked by distinct reporting milestones. Each insurer is required to report to the MAIC when key milestone events (Notification, Compliance, Liability, Settlement, Finalisation) have occurred. A high-level process map is show in Fig. 3. The Act lays down maximum periods for determining whether the claim is compliant with the Act and the insurer(s) that is/are liable for the claim. (*NB* where more than one insurer is deemed liable for the claim, one insurer will be designated responsible for managing the claim.) Following the establishment of liability, the managing insurer will process the claim till finalisation. Following the liability stage, the progress of the claim is determined by factors such as (i) all parties agreeing that the injured person has reached a stage of *maximum medical stability* beyond which further recovery will not occur, (ii) the insurer and claimant agreeing a settlement offer, or (iii) mediation or litigation determining a settlement. In our case study, we considered 4,959 claims managed by one of the commercial CTP insurers comprising cases that were 'open' at some stage in the period 1-Jan-2012 to 17-Oct-2015 (3,446 'closed' claims and 1,513 'open' claims at time of data extract). The event log itself comprises 1,982,009 event records extracted from various components of the insurer's claims management system including documents, notes, automated/system generated tasks, user initiated activities, records of changes to a claim's compliance status and records of damages estimates generated at various points in a claims history. The event log also contained events representing CTP scheme milestone dates. Overall, there were 180 different activity codes.

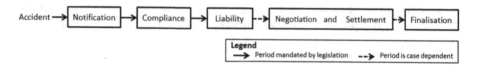

Fig. 3. Reporting milestones in the CTP claims management process

An initial analysis of the event log revealed a pattern of 'batch completion' of assigned tasks by system users. That is, the insurer's claims management system presents a user with a set of tasks ordered by due date. The user may select and mark as 'completed' one or more tasks at a time. Further, the insurer's claims management system is a workflow management system which will generate tasks for users based on the current state of claims processing. More than one task may be generated at the same time. The batch completion and multi-task generation pose some problems in quantifying shelf time in any given claim.

Here we note that in the event log, the start time of an activity was the date/time on which the task was assigned to a user. The complete time for an activity was the date/time when the user marked the task as 'completed'. **NB.** *It was not possible to determine, from the data available, when the user first started working on the task. That is, it was not possible to determine the period between the date/time the task was assigned to the user and the date/time the user first started working on the task. Nor was it possible to determine whether the user worked continuously on the task or completed the task in installments.*

Table 1. Shelf time instances and distribution by claim status. Periods of shelf time were deemed to be significant if they exceeded 340 h (approx 2 weeks).

Claim status	Total shelf time periods	# Claims	Significant shelf time periods	# Claims
Closed	14,336	3,014	2,832	1,178
Open	8,280	1,481	2,385	1,279
Totals	22,617	4,495	5,217	3,057

Our initial analysis revealed that periods of shelf time were common in the claims under consideration. Table 1 shows the numbers of shelf time periods by claim status. It can be seen that across the entire corpus of claims, more than 60% of claims (3,057 of 4,959 claims) were affected by at least one significant shelf time period ($\theta = 340$ h). Figure 4 shows, for the 2,939 claims where total shelf time exceeded 680 h (1 month), the fraction of the claim comprising of shelf time.

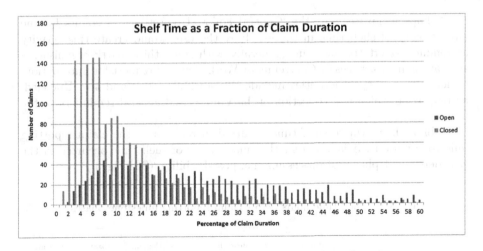

Fig. 4. Shelf time as a fraction of claim duration

Table 2 shows the top 10 activities that most heavily impact on shelf time hours.

Table 2. Activities triggering shelf time periods

Code	Label	Total shelf hrs	Instances	Avg hrs per instance	Distinct cases	Avg case frequency	Avg shelf hrs per case
CTP_10_011	General follow up activity	2, 310, 990	5, 480	422	2, 947	1.9	784
rm_ap_review assigndoc category	Review and assign category to new document	774, 919	3, 049	254	1, 653	1.8	469
CTP_10_008	Interim coding	702, 130	1, 278	549	1, 047	1.2	671
CTP_02_011	Review and update claim estimates and quantum	563, 813	808	698	734	1.1	768
CTP_90_011	Review and action new statutory bodies document	522, 741	862	606	700	1.2	747
CTP_01_019	Review claim for fraud potential	374, 056	901	415	692	1.3	541
CTP_90_002	Review and action new correspondence document	357, 539	1, 647	217	1, 046	1.6	342
CTP_10_005	Action invoice/cheque	314, 912	1, 430	220	1, 050	1.4	300
CTP_03_007	Rehab follow up	243, 248	256	950	236	1.1	1, 031
Uncoded	Assorted follow ups	228, 331	604	378	503	1.2	454

Perhaps unsurprisingly, the 'General Follow Up Activity' accounts for the largest block of shelf time in the log. Here the user would create this activity as reminder/alert to follow up (generally with some third party organisation such as medical services or Centrelink or Work Cover) a request for information. Other follow up type activities include 'Rehab Follow Up' and the 'Uncoded' activity code which is a collection of diary notes and general reminders to the user.

Table 3 shows where shelf time occurred in relation to the claim reporting milestone periods. It is apparent that most hours of shelf time occurred in the case-dependent phases of processing, i.e. post-Liability. (See Fig. 3.)

Table 3. Shelf time hours across claim reporting milestone phases

Code	Label	Post-notification	Post-compliance	Post-liability	Post-settlement	Post-finalisation	Code total shelf hrs
CTP_10_011	General follow up activity	68,871	119,397	1,629,414	461,731	31,577	2,310,990
rm_ap_revi-ewassigndoc category	Review and assign category to new document	17,138	43,138	336,429	135,885	242,329	774,919
CTP_10_008	Interim coding	8,638	23,668	308,676	325,481	35,667	702,130
CTP_02_011	Review and update claim estimates and quantum	20,768	4,373	389,374	142,668	6,630	563,813
CTP_90_011	Review and action new statutory bodies document	6,628	10,162	63,912	53,593	388,446	522,741
CTP_01_019	Review claim for fraud potential	15,061	19,562	276,287	63,131	15	374,056
CTP_90_002	Review and action new correspon-dence document	12,348	34,414	211,259	33,966	65,552	357,539
CTP_10_005	Action Invoice/Cheque	5,513	8,583	74,256	106,828	119,732	314,912
CTP_03_007	Rehab follow up	793	11,387	217,962	8,284	4,822	243,248
Uncoded	Assorted follow ups	2,039	3,989	139,385	82,916	2	228,331

The case study findings showed that individual instances of shelf time (period greater than 2 weeks) occurred in 62% of all claims and that 59% of all claims experienced total shelf time of greater than 1 month. The technique was able to identify activities that triggered a period of shelf time and to quantify the total shelf time frequency and durations associated with each activity/trigger. The technique was also able to identify shelf time periods across the different phases (sub-processes) of the CTP insurance claim process which showed that, in general, the phase associated with most shelf time is the Post-Liability phase. We do note, however, some interesting observations including the large number of shelf time hours associated with the rm_ap_reviewassigndoccategory and CTP_90_011 activity codes in the Post-Finalisation phase. These will form the basis for further investigation in conjunction with the process stakeholder.

5   Conclusion

An understanding of shelf time (idle time that exceeds some process-dependent threshold) provide insights to process behaviour and acts as input to process improvement strategies. In this paper we have described a process mining-based technique suitable for identifying and quantifying shelf time in an event log. The technique takes an event log extracted from historical executions of a business process and requires each event in the log to have timestamps that can be used to represent the start and completion of the event. The essence of the shelf time identification technique is finding events which do not temporally 'overlap' other events in the same case in the log. The approach has been applied to a real-life event log extracted from a major, commercial, Queensland CTP insurer. Finally, the technique is robust enough to use event attributes other than the activity label that trigger shelf time periods. For instance, it would be possible to determine shelf time periods associated with the resource assigned to an event.

Acknowledgements. The research for this article was supported by a Queensland Government Accelerate Partnerships grant. We gratefully acknowledge the contributions made to this project by Neil Singleton (Insurance Commissioner). We would also like to thank the stakeholders of the commercial insurer for their time and valuable contributions to this work.

References

1. van der Aalst, W.M.P., et al.: Process mining manifesto. In: Daniel, F., Barkaoui, K., Dustdar, S. (eds.) BPM 2011. LNBIP, vol. 99, pp. 169–194. Springer, Heidelberg (2012). doi:10.1007/978-3-642-28108-2_19
2. Fetter, R.B., Thompson, J.D.: Patients' waiting time and doctors' idle time in the outpatient setting. Health Serv. Res. 1(1), 66 (1966)
3. Mans, R., Schonenberg, M., Leonardi, G., Panzarasa, S., Cavallini, A., Quaglini, S., van der Aalst, W.: Process mining techniques: an application to stroke care. In: Ehealth Beyond the Horizon- Get it There (2008)
4. Partington, A., Wynn, M.T., Suriadi, S., Ouyang, C., Karnon, J.: Process mining for clinical processes: a comparative analysis of four Australian hospitals. ACM Trans. Manag. Inf. Syst. 5(4), 19:1–19:18 (2015). http://doi.acm.org/10.1145/2629446
5. Rai, P., Trivedi, R., Nath, R.: Cycle time and idle time analysis of draglines for increased productivity-a case study. Indian J. Eng. Mater. Sci. 7(2), 77–81 (2000)
6. Rozinat, A., de Jong, I.S., Günther, C.W., van der Aalst, W.M.: Process mining applied to the test process of wafer scanners in ASML. IEEE Trans. Syst. Man Cybern. Part C (Applications and Reviews) 39(4), 474–479 (2009)

7. Suriadi, S., Andrews, R., ter Hofstede, A.H., Wynn, M.T.: Event log imperfection patterns for process mining: towards a systematic approach to cleaning event logs. Inform. Syst. **64**, 132–150 (2017)
8. Suriadi, S., Ouyang, C., van der Aalst, W.M., ter Hofstede, A.H.: Event interval analysis: why do processes take time? Decis. Support Syst. **79**, 77–98 (2015)
9. Suriadi, S., Wynn, M.T., Ouyang, C., ter Hofstede, A.H.M., van Dijk, N.J.: Understanding process behaviours in a large insurance company in Australia: a case study. In: Salinesi, C., Norrie, M.C., Pastor, Ó. (eds.) CAiSE 2013. LNCS, vol. 7908, pp. 449–464. Springer, Heidelberg (2013). doi:10.1007/978-3-642-38709-8_29
10. Yoo, S., Cho, M., Kim, E., Kim, S., Sim, Y., Yoo, D.H., Hwang, H., Song, M.: Assessment of hospital processes using a process mining technique: outpatient process analysis at a tertiary hospital. Int. J. Med. Inform. **88**, 34–43 (2016). http://dx.doi.org/10.1016/j.ijmedinf.2015.12.018
11. Zou, J., Kim, H.: Using hue, saturation, and value color space for hydraulic excavator idle time analysis. J. Comput. Civil Eng. **21**(4), 238–246 (2007)

Automated Product-Attribute Mapping

Karamjit Singh, Garima Gupta$^{(\boxtimes)}$, Gautam Shroff, and Puneet Agarwal

TCS Research, Gurgaon 122003, India
{karamjit.singh,gupta.garima1,gautam.shroff,puneet.a}@tcs.com

Abstract. Aggregate analysis, such as comparing country-wise sales versus global market share across product categories, is often complicated by the unavailability of common join attributes, e.g., category, across diverse datasets from different geographies or retail chains. Sometimes this is a missing data issue, while in other cases it may be inherent, e.g., the records in different geographical databases may actually describe different product 'SKUs', or follow different norms for categorization. Often a tedious manual mapping process is often employed in practice. We focus on improving such a process using machine-learning driven automation. Record linkage techniques, such as [5] can be used to automatically map products in different data sources to a common set of *global* attributes, thereby enabling federated aggregation joins to be performed. Traditional record-linkage techniques are typically unsupervised, relying textual similarity features across attributes to estimate matches. In this paper, we present an ensemble model combining minimal supervision using Bayesian network models together with unsupervised textual matching for automating such 'attribute fusion'. We present results of our approach on a large volume of real-life data from a market-research scenario and compare with a standard record matching algorithm. Our approach is especially suited for practical implementation since we also provide confidence values for matches, enabling routing of items for human intervention where required.

1 Introduction

In most large enterprises the process of generation of business reports that fuse and aggregate data from multiple sources leads to a number of challenges; for example, dealing with incongruous join keys between different datasets. Even if a machine-learning based data fusion method is adopted for partially automating such matchings, there remains another challenge of how to imbibe the new approach in the main-stream business process so as to enable human intervention when accurate automation is not possible.

We focus on one such process that is widely applicable to many enterprises, and propose business process improvement utilizing the machine-learning and data-mining based methods which follows 'human-in-the-loop' paradigm with enhanced efficiency. Manufacturers as well as retailers often need to analyze product performance reports based on the data received from multiple geographies (see Fig. 3), about measures such as sales volume and revenue along dimensions such as brand-name and product segment. Unfortunately, the terms used

© Springer International Publishing AG 2017
U Kang et al. (Eds.): PAKDD 2017 Workshops, LNAI 10526, pp. 163–175, 2017.
DOI: 10.1007/978-3-319-67274-8_15

to describe the same attribute of a product are different in every geography, necessitating some matching procedure, which is often manually done in practice. Further, due to introduction of new retail chains, and new products in the retail market, this is a never ending continuous process.

The goal of such a process is to fuse information about consumer products, such as sales, market share, etc., which is spread across disparate databases belonging to different organizations, in which each product is *not* identifiable via a common key. For example, a *Global database (DB)* might track overall market-share of global product categories. On the other hand, each *Local DB* might track sales data within geographies using local-product-ids along with other characteristics, but *not* the global category-id. As a result, an analytical task such as comparing the sales of product categories within each geography against their global market share becomes difficult due to the lack of a natural join attribute between the databases.

Process Overview: *Local DB* contains attributes that can help to identify/classify the product that a particular record measures. For example, in case of carbonated drinks, each record usually contains attributes such as brand, flavor, material used etc. However, these attributes are inconsistent across geographies: The same product could be defined using different values of attributes across different countries and different retailers. Figure 1, shows an example in which values of four attributes (shown in first column) are different for the same product across four different countries. Additionally, *Local DB* may also contain textual *description* of products entered manually by retailers. Figure 2 shows such descriptions for the same product from different retailers. Number of descriptions of a single product in one geography may go upto the order of hundreds.

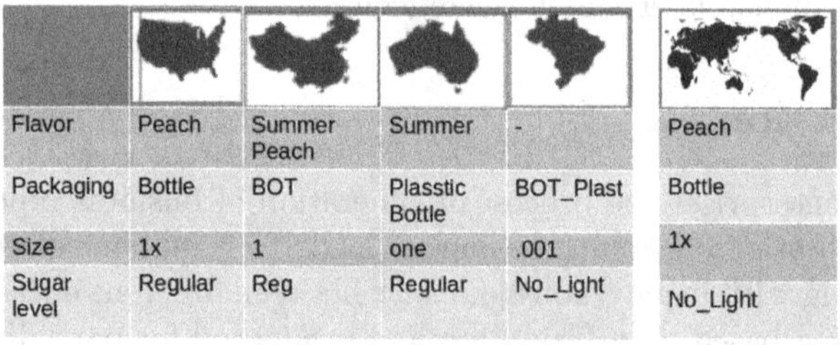

Flavor	Peach	Summer Peach	Summer	-	Peach
Packaging	Bottle	BOT	Plasstic Bottle	BOT_Plast	Bottle
Size	1x	1	one	.001	1x
Sugar level	Regular	Reg	Regular	No_Light	No_Light

Fig. 1. *Local DB* showing local attributes of the same product across four geographies and their corresponding global attributes

One way to perform analysis across disparate databases is by mapping records in each *Local DB* to their corresponding global attributes (e.g., right most column of Fig. 2). However, preparing such mappings is a huge manual and complicated task because: (a) The cardinality (number of possible values) of local and global characteristics varies from tens to thousands, and (b) Uncertainty in

Item	Retailer Description
XXXX	WILD CHERRY BRAND 12PK CHERRY
XXXX	BRAND WCHERR!
XXXX	WLD CD BRAND 12PK
XXXX	WILD CHERRY BRAND 12 PK CAN-0144000(OZ)

Fig. 2. Five different retailer descriptions of the same product. Actual brand name is hidden to maintain client confidentiality.

the semantics of local characteristics of the same product from different geographies, leading to confusion in identifying the product category, even by human annotators.

Our aim is to help reduce cost of the operational process of creating and maintaining such global references by reducing manual workload via automation via modern data-lake architecture that include automated fusion of federated databases. Our goal is to either make high confidence predictions, or abstain from making any prediction so that such records can be sent to human annotators. We want to minimize the number of such abstentions while maximizing the precision of the predictions.

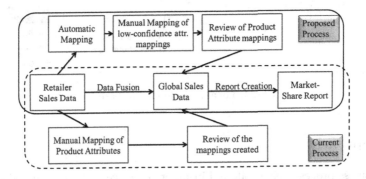

Fig. 3. Current and Modified/Proposed Product attribute matching process

Attribute Fusion using Record Matching: Consider two databases (see Fig. 4): (a) *Local DB(L)* of a single geography with each product l having local characteristics $L_1, L_2, ..., L_M$, e.g., flavor, brand, etc., and retailer descriptions (D_l), and (b) a *Global DB(G)* having K global characteristics. The problem at hand is thus a *record matching* problem where products in local database are to be mapped to global characteristic values (e.g. 'category', or 'global brand' etc.).

Note that our objective is only to reconcile performance metrics (such as volume sales and market-share) across databases for each global characteristic *independently*, e.g., sales vs market-share for each category, or alternatively each global brand, etc. We can achieve this by solving K different record matching problems, as shown in Fig. 4: For each product, we shall predict each of the K global characteristics given local characteristics and retailer descriptions separately, as $\arg\max_j P(G_j|L_1, ..., L_M, D_l)$.

In this paper: (a) We address the problem of automating attribute fusion across diverse data sources that do not share a common join key. (b) We augment traditional, fundamentally unsupervised text-similarly techniques with supervised, Bayesian network models in a confidence-based ensemble for automating the mapping process. (c) Our approach additionally delivers confidence bounds on its predictions, so that human annotation can be employed when needed and business process could be improved. (d) We test our approach in a real-life market research scenario. We also compare it with available techniques [5] and demonstrate that our approach outperforms FEBRL [5]. (e) We illustrate how our approach has been integrated into a data-fusion platform [17] specifically designed to manage data-lakes containing disparate databases.

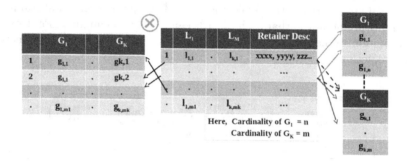

Fig. 4. Local and global database

2   Approach

The business process being followed in practice, as well as the modified process is shown in Fig. 3. In the current process all local products from local database need to be mapped to global product list. We propose to predict the global characteristics of local product list using machine-learning and data-mining based approach, along with a prediction confidence measure. Based on this confidence measure a choice is made about which of the automatically performed characteristic mappings should be discarded, and mapped manually. This leads to reduction in manual effort and increased efficiency of business process.

Further from the data-mining point of view, each product l in L has two kind of information (1) M Local characteristics and (2) Textual descriptions by retailers. In this section, we present our approach to predict the value of global characteristic G_j for each product in L. We use two different models for two different datasets (1) Supervised Bayesian Model (SBM) using local characteristics, and (2) Unsupervised Textual Similarity (UTS) using descriptions to compute probability of every possible state $g_{j,t}, t = 1, 2, ..., m_j$ of G_j. Finally, we use an weighted ensemble based approach to combine the probabilities of both models to predict the value of G_j.

2.1   Supervised Bayesian Model

Approach to build SBM comprises of: (1) Network Structure Learning, (2) Parameter Learning, & (3) Bayesian Inference. For structure learning, we propose a novel technique of learning Tree based Bayesian Networks (TBN), whereas for parameter learning and Bayesian inference, we use the idea of [21] that performs probabilistic queries using SQL queries on the database of conditional probability tables.

TBN Structure Learning: Bayesian networks are associated with parameters known as conditional probability tables (CPT), where a CPT of a node indicates the probability that each value of a node can take given all combinations of values of its parent nodes. In CPTs, the number of bins grows exponentially as the number of parents increases leaving fewer data instances in each bin for estimating the parameters. Thus, sparser structures often provide better estimation of the underlying distribution [10]. Also, if the number of states of each node becomes high and the learned model is complex, Bayesian inferencing becomes conceptually and computationally intractable [12]. Hence, tree-based structures can be useful for density estimation from limited data and in the presence of higher number of states for facilitating faster inferencing. We employ a greedy search, and score based approach for learning TBN structure.

Given the global characteristic G_j and M local characteristics, we find set of top η most relevant local characteristics w.r.t. G_j using mutual information. We denote these η local characteristics by the set $Y^j(L)$. Further, we learn a *Tree based Bayesian Network (TBN)* on random variables $X = \{X_r : r = 1, 2, ..., \eta + 1\}$, where each $X_r \in X$ is either local characteristic $L_i \in Y^j(L)$ or global characteristic G_j

Chow et al. in [4] state that cross-entropy between the tree structures distributions and the actual underlying distribution is minimized when the structure is a maximum weight spanning tree (MST). So, in order to learn TBN structure, we first learn MST for the characteristics in the set X. We find the mutual information between each pair characteristics, denoted by $W(X_r, X_s)$. Further, we use the mutual information as the weight between each pair of characteristics and learn MST using Kruskal's algorithm.

$$TotalWeight(TW) = \sum_{r=1, Pa(X_r) \neq 0}^{\eta+1} W(X_r, Pa(X_r)) \qquad (1)$$

By learning MST, order of search space of possible graphs is reduced to $2^{O(\eta)}$, from $2^{O((\eta)^2)}$. Using this MST, we search for the directed graph with least cross-entropy, by flipping each edge directions sequentially to obtain 2^η directed graphs along with their corresponding *Totel weight (TW)* calculated using Eq. 1.

Graph with maximum TW (minimum cross-entropy) [12] is chosen as the best graphical structure representative of underlying distribution.

Parameter Learning and Inference: To learn the parameters (CPTs) of Bayesian Network, for every product l in L we compute the probabilities $p_{j,1}^l, p_{j,2}^l, ..., p_{j,m_j}^l$, for every state of G_j, given the observed values of local characteristics in the Bayesian network, using an approach described in [21]. Here, CPTs are learned from the data stored in RDBMS and all queries are also answered using SQL.

2.2   Unsupervised Text Similarity

In this section, we present UTS approach to compute the probability $q_{j,1}^l, q_{j,2}^l, ...,$ q_{j,m_j}^l of each possible state of the global characteristic G_j using retailer descriptions. Consider each product l in L has r_l descriptions and for each description $d_{l,r}$, where $r = 1, 2, ..., r_l$, we find n-grams of adjacent words. Let $N_l = \{n_v^l, v = 1, 2, ...\}$ be the set of n-grams of all descriptions, where f_v^l be the frequency of each n_v^l defined as a ratio of the number of descriptions in which n_v^l exists to the r_l.

For every state $g_{j,t}$ of G_j, we find the best matching n-gram from the set N_l by calculating Jaro-Wrinkler distance between $g_{j,t}$ and every $n_v^l \in N_l$ and choose the n-gram, say $n_{v,t}^l$, with the maximum score $s_{j,t}^l$. Further, multiply the scores $s_{j,t}^l$ with the frequency of $n_{v,t}^l$ to get the new score i.e., $S_{j,t}^l = s_{j,t}^l \times f_{l,t}^s$. Finally, we convert each score $S_{j,t}^l$ into the probability $q_{j,t}^l$ by using softmax scaling function.

2.3   Ensemble of Models

In ensemble approach, we first find confidence of each prediction in both the cases (SBM and UTS) and then use these confidence values as weights for weighted ensemble. Given the probability distribution $\{p_{j,t}^l : t = 1, 2, ..., m_j\}$ for the values of G_j using SBM model, we find the confidence corresponds to each probability as

$$C(p_{j,t}^l) = 1 - \sqrt{\sum_{t'=1}^{m_j} (p_{j,t'}^l - h_{t'}^l(t))^2}, t = 1, 2..., m_j \tag{2}$$

where $h_{t'}^l(t)$ is the ideal distribution, which is 1 when $t = t'$ and 0 otherwise. Similarly, we can find the confidence $C(q_{j,t}^l)$ of each probability $q_{j,t}^l$.

With the given probability distribution and the confidence values from both models, we take weighted linear sum of two probabilities to get the new probability distribution over the states of G_j: $P_{j,t}^l = C(p_{j,t}^l) \times p_{j,t}^l + C(q_{j,t}^l) \times q_{j,t}^l, t = 1, 2, ..., m_j$ and we choose the value of G_j for maximum $P_{j,t}^l$.

CoP: For every prediction, we assign the confidence value called confidence of prediction (CoP). CoP is a measure that helps to decide whether the predicted value is trustworthy or not. Given the probability distribution $\{P_{j,t}^l : l = 1, 2, ..., m_j\}$ for the values of g_j, we calculate the CoP of the predicted value $g_{j,t}^l$ of G_j by using Eq. 2.

3   Experiments and Results

We present the accuracy of our predictions on a real-life dataset from a global
market research organization. We set a threshold τ on CoP, and predictions with
a CoP $< \tau$ are routed for human annotation. We also measure the accuracies of
our predictions for different values of τ.

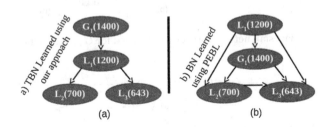

Fig. 5. Structure learned of G_1 using two different approaches

Data Description: We have data for carbonated drinks of 26K unique
products from a single geography, contained in two datasets: (a) **Local DB**: It
contains 26 K products with each product having 49 local characteristics, where
cardinality of local characteristics varies from tens to thousands. It also contains descriptions of products given by retailers of that product, where number
of descriptions of a single product varies from tens to hundreds. (b) **Global
DB**: It contains four global characteristics with cardinality varying from tens to
thousands.

Data Preparation: We predict four global characteristics G_1, G_2, G_3, and
G_4 for two cases, with varying ratio of split between training, validation and test
datasets. ***Case-1*** (60:20:20) has 60% training, 20% validation and 20% test and
Case-2 has this ratio as 20:20:60. **NOTE:** While Case-1 uses a traditional split
of training vs testing data, Case-2 is more realistic, since in practice preparing
a training data by manual data labeling is costly: For example, we would like to
'onboard' a data from a particular dataset by manually annotating only a small
fraction (e.g. 20%) of records and automate the remainder or we might like
to board data from one organization (e.g. retailer or distributor) in a particular
geography in the hope that data from remaining sources in that geography share
similar local characteristics, eliminating manual annotation for a large volume
of data. To simulate this practical scenario, we used the first few records from
the local dataset, which happened to contain only 10% or so of the total possible
values of each global attribute.

For SBM, η relevant local characteristics was chosen for every G_j. Figure 5,
compares the TBN structure learned using our approach and another learned
using an open source python library Pebl [16], for the global characteristic G_1.
Clearly, network obtained using Pebl (Fig. 5(b)) is more complex as compared
to ours 5(a), as the size of CPTs of these are of the order of (a) 1200×1400 and

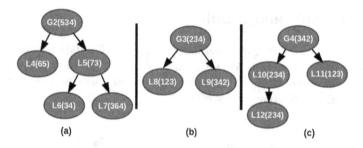

Fig. 6. Tree based Bayesian network structures learned for G_2, G_3, G_4 global attributes.

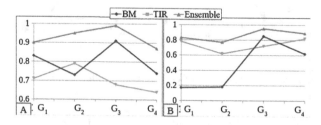

Fig. 7. x-axis: global characteristics, y-axis: (A) Predictive accuracy for Case-1, (B) Predictive accuracy for Case-2

(b) $1200 \times 1400 \times 700 \times 643$ respectively. Figure 6 shows the Bayesian network structure learned for the remaining three global attributes (G_2, G_3, G_4).

Figure 7, shows the prediction accuracy of four global characteristic for Case-1 and Case-2 respectively. Here, the accuracy is a ratio of correctly predicted products to the total number of products. In Case-1, accuracy of Ensemble model is in the range of 85 to 99% and it outperforms both SBM and UTS for all four global characteristics. Case-2 (Fig. 7-B), naturally renders the SBM less accurate, since the training data contains only 10% of possible states of each global characteristic. However, it is compensated by the performance of UTS, which searches the target set of global attribute values from the retailer descriptions. Combining these models using our Ensemble model the accuracy of four global characteristics reaches 78 to 93%.

Baseline Comparison: We also compared our approach with record matching method implemented in a framework called FEBRL [5]. In FEBRL, we consider two databases (1) Local DB with the products having local characteristics and corresponding retailer descriptions, (2) Global DB having all possible values of a single global characteristic. The problem statement is to match products in local DB to the Global DB. For attribute matching, we tried three similarity measures winkler, tokenset, trigam and show the results with winkler which outperforms the rest. We tested this approach for the Case-1 on the smaller dataset (5K products) for all four global characteristics separately. Table 1, shows the comparison of the prediction accuracy of four global attributes using our Ensemble approach and FEBRL. In case of FEBRL, prediction accuracy is the number of correctly matched products out of all products in local DB. This suggests that our approach outperforms and also shows that accuracy of FEBRL decreases for high cardinality global attributes. FEBRL did not work on, 26k products, on a machine with 16 GB RAM, Intel Core i7-3520M CPU 2.90 GHz* 4, 64 bit. We did not try the blocking method as main motive of our problem is to improve accuracy of prediction, and not the time complexity.

Table 1. Comparison of our approach with FEBRL

Global att	Num of states	FEBRL(winkler)	Ensemble
G_1	107	86%	93%
G_2	154	57%	95.2%
G_3	3	99.3%	99.2%
G_4	13	95.4%	99.4%

CoP Threshold for human annotation: We define three categories: (a) **P-C:** Number of products *predicted correctly* by our approach for which CoP $> \tau$. (b) **P-I:** Number of products *predicted incorrectly*, for which CoP $> \tau$. (c) **NP:** Products which we choose *not to predict*, i.e., products with CoP $\leq \tau$. We select τ in order to maximize P-C and minimize P-I category, while not increasing NP so much that exercise becomes almost entirely manual. Since products in the P-I category are more costly for a company as compared to NP category, we give more weight to P-I while learning τ. Table 2, shows the percentage of products in each category (P-C, P-I, NP) on validation set along with the threshold τ values for both cases. It shows that for given τ, percentage of products in P-C category is in the range of 81–96% for Case-1, whereas, it ranges from 70 to 96% for Case-2. Also, the average percentage of products in P-I category is only around 5%. These numbers establish that CoP is a good measure for reliability of predictions. Figure 8, shows the variation in the percentage of products in test set of each category with respect to threshold value τ for both Case-1 and Case-2, for the global characteristic G_1. It validates the optimal values of τ learned using validation set, 0.5 for Case-1 and 0.6 for Case-2.

Table 2. Percentage of products in each category on validation set

Global	Case-1				Case-2			
	τ	P-C	P-I	NP	τ	P-C	P-I	NP
G_1	0.5	92%	4%	4%	0.6	82%	7%	11%
G_2	0.6	81%	7%	12%	0.65	74%	10%	16%
G_3	0.7	96%	1%	3%	0.7	96%	1%	3%
G_4	0.8	86%	3%	11%	0.8	85%	4%	11%

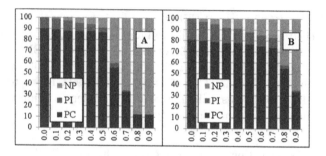

Fig. 8. % of Products in each category for different values of τ on test data for G_1 in (A) Case-1 and (B) Case-2

The process of aggregate analysis, comparing global market share and sales of product categories is carried out in our platform *iFuse* [17] (Fig. 9). Figure 9(a) and (b) shows the data tile and cart view of iFuse representing the attributes of the local DB and global DB to be linked together. Figure 9(c) shows the tile view of the attributes obtained after mapping of local DB to global attribute, here GLO BRAND via ensemble approach, thereby enabling the **join** of local sales and global market share via common global attribute, GLO BRAND (Fig. 9(d)). Figure 9(e) shows aggregate analysis of different products via motionchart.

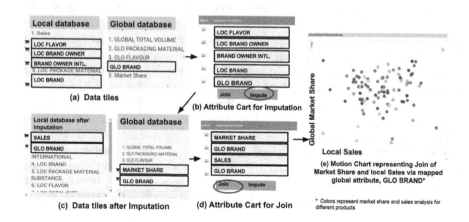

Fig. 9. Figure showing aggregate analysis of global market share and local sales done using our platform.

4   Related Work

Record linkage of entities across disparate datasets is a widely explored [3], which has been applied in wide variety of domains like environmental hazards [1], drug safety [14], and to different types of data, including text [13] and images [9].

While record linkage addresses the problem of extracting, matching and resolving entities in structured and unstructured data [8] across disparate datasets, with or without join keys, our problem address different aspect of record linkage *where disparate databases need to be fused in the absence of natural join key*.

Record linkage problem has been addressed generally via two category of approaches, learning based and non-learning based [11]. Learning based approaches include FEBRL [5] which uses support vector machine (SVM) for learning suitable matcher combinations, and MARLIN (Multiply Adaptive Record Linkage with Induction) [2] which uses two string similarity measures (Edit Distance and Cosine) and several learners, specifically SVM and decision trees. In non-learning based approaches, PPJoin+ [20] is a single-attribute match approach (similarity join) using sophisticated filtering techniques for improved efficiency, and FellegiSunter [6] evaluates three of the similarity measures provided by FEBRL (Winkler, Tokenset, Trigram) and has an lower and upper similarity threshold that can be adjusted. In [15], an ensemble approach of two non-learning algorithms Fellegi-Sunter (FS) and Jaro-Wrinkler (JW) has been presented for record-linkage. In contrast, we use confidence based ensemble approach that combines learning based Bayesian model and a non-learning based textual model. Our approach also produces confidence bound on the predictions that help to decide reliability of prediction.

Bayesian Networks are used for modeling beliefs in various domains like bioinformatics [7], medicine [19], manufacturing [18]. While traditional approximate inference techniques for Bayesian graphical modeling are able to deal with larger networks, they are usually restricted to models with low cardinalities of attributes. In our approach of BGM, we handle high cardinality attributes by introducing a novel approach of learning restricted Tree based Bayesian network, which facilitates faster (exact) inferencing. Our work in BGM is closest to [21], which presents an approach to compute distributional queries by approximating the underlying joint distribution via a Bayesian network. In [21], SQL database has been used for Bayesian inferencing under the assumption of simple networks, which are learned entirely using domain knowledge. In our work of BGM, we present end to end approach of Bayesian graphical modeling which learns simple tree based structure followed by exact Bayesian inferencing accelerated by an SQL engine to predict global characteristics.

5 Conclusion

We have addressed a particular class of record-linkage problems where disparate databases need to be fused in the absence of matching keys for the limited purpose of aggregate analysis. Our ensemble approach combines supervised Bayesian models with unsupervised textual similarity, and also returns confidence along with each prediction. We submit that our approach is likely to be applicable for similar instances of record-linkage in a wide variety of applications, even while attempting to fuse data from external sources, such as social media, sensor data etc. Such scenarios are becoming increasingly common as the *data lake* para-digm is gradually replacing the traditional data-warehouse model, driven by the availability and accessibility of external 'big data' sources.

References

1. Acheson, E., Peto, R.: Record linkage and the identification of long-term environmental hazards [and discussion]. Proc. Roy. Soc. London B Biol. Sci. **205**, 165–178 (1979)
2. Bilenko, M., Mooney, R.J.: Adaptive duplicate detection using learnable string similarity measures. In: ACM SIGKDD International Conference on Knowledge Discovery and Data Mining. ACM (2003)
3. Brizan, D.G., Tansel, A.U.: A survey of entity resolution and record linkage methodologies. Commun. IIMA **6**, 5 (2015)
4. Chow, C., Liu, C.: Approximating discrete probability distributions with dependence trees. IEEE Trans. Inf. Theory **14**, 462–467 (1968)
5. Christen, P.: Febrl: a freely available record linkage system with a graphical user interface. In: 2nd Australasian Workshop on Health Data and Knowledge Management, vol. 80. Australian Computer Society, Inc. (2008)
6. Fellegi, I.P., Sunter, A.B.: A theory for record linkage. J. Am. Stat. Assoc. **64**, 1183–1210 (1969)
7. Friedman, N., Linial, M., Nachman, I., Pe'er, D.: Using bayesian networks to analyze expression data. J. Comput. Biol. **7**, 601–620 (2000)
8. Getoor, L., Machanavajjhala, A.: Entity resolution: theory, practice & open challenges. Proc. VLDB Endow. **5**, 2018–2019 (2012)
9. Huang, T., Russell, S.: Object identification: a bayesian analysis with application to traffic surveillance. Artif. Intell. **103**, 77–93 (1998)
10. Koller, D., Friedman, N.: Probabilistic Graphical Models: Principles and Techniques. MIT press, Cambridge (2009)
11. Köpcke, H., Thor, A., Rahm, E.: Evaluation of entity resolution approaches on real-world match problems. Proc. VLDB Endow. **3**, 484–493 (2010)
12. Lam, W., Bacchus, F.: Learning bayesian belief networks: an approach based on the MDL principle. Comput. Intell. **10**, 269–293 (1994)
13. Li, X., Morie, P., Roth, D.: Semantic integration in text: from ambiguous names to identifiable entities. AI Mag. **26**, 45 (2005)
14. Norén, G.N., Orre, R., Bate, A.: A hit-miss model for duplicate detection in the who drug safety database. In: Proceedings of the Eleventh ACM SIGKDD International Conference on Knowledge Discovery in Data Mining. ACM (2005)
15. Poon, S., Poon, J., Lam, M., et al.: An ensemble approach for record matching in data linkage. Stud. Health Technol. Inf. **227**, 113–119 (2016)
16. Shah, A., Woolf, P.: Python environment for bayesian learning: inferring the structure of bayesian networks from knowledge and data. J. Mach. Learn. Res. JMLR **10**, 159–162 (2009)
17. Singh, K., Paneri, et al.: Visual bayesian fusion to navigate a data lake. In: 2016 19th International Conference on Information Fusion (FUSION). ISIF (2016)
18. Singh, K., Shroff, G., Agarwal, P.: Predictive reliability mining for early warnings in populations of connected machines. In: IEEE International Conference on Data Science and Advanced Analytics (DSAA). 36678 2015. IEEE (2015)

19. Uebersax, J.: Genetic Counseling and Cancer Risk Modeling: An Application of Bayes Nets. Ravenpack International, Marbella (2004)
20. Xiao, C., Wang, W., Lin, X., Yu, J.X., Wang, G.: Efficient similarity joins for near-duplicate detection. ACM Trans. Database Syst
21. Yadav, S., Shroff, G., Hassan, E., Agarwal, P.: Business data fusion. In: 2015 18th International Conference on Information Fusion (Fusion). IEEE (2015)

A Novel Extreme Learning Machine-Based Classification Algorithm for Uncertain Data

Xianchao Zhang[1], Daoyuan Sun[1], Yuangang Li[2,3], Han Liu[1], and Wenxin Liang[1(✉)]

[1] School of Software Technology, Dalian University of Technology, Dalian 116620, China
{xczhang,wxliang}@dlut.edu.cn, amossdy@mail.dlut.edu.cn, liu.han.dut@gmail.com
[2] Shanghai University of Finance and Economics, Shanghai 200433, China
[3] Goldpac Limited, Zhuhai 519070, China
gary.li@goldpac.com

Abstract. Traditional classification algorithms are widely used on determinate data. However, uncertain data is ubiquitous in many real applications, which poses a great challenge to traditional classification algorithms. Extreme learning machine (ELM) is a traditional and powerful classification algorithm. However, existing ELM-based uncertain data classification algorithms can not deal with data uncertainty well. In this paper, we propose a novel ELM-based uncertain data classification algorithm, called UELM. UELM firstly employs exact probability density function (PDF) instead of expected values or sample points to model uncertain data, thus avoiding the loss of uncertain information (probability distribution information of uncertain data). Furthermore, UELM redesigns the traditional ELM algorithm by modifying the received content of input layer and the activation function of hidden layer, thus making the ELM algorithm more applicable to uncertain data. Extensive experimental results on different datasets show that our proposed UELM algorithm outperforms the baselines in accuracy and efficiency.

Keywords: Extreme learning machine · Uncertain data · Classification

1 Introduction

Classification is one of the important problems in machine learning and data mining [12]. Traditional classification algorithms are based on the assumption that the input data are determinate. However, data uncertainty is ubiquitous in many real scenarios. For example, in the data mining applications of Business Process Management (BPM), customers evaluate a commodity by scoring on various aspects, such as quality, performance and user friendliness. Each commodity may be scored by many customers. Thus, the customer satisfaction to a

This work was supported by 863 project of China (No. 2015AA015403) and NSFC (No. 61632019).

U Kang et al. (Eds.): PAKDD 2017 Workshops, LNAI 10526, pp. 176–188, 2017.
DOI: 10.1007/978-3-319-67274-8_16

commodity can be modeled as an uncertain object on the customer score space. The market manager can make decisions according to customer satisfaction data. If data uncertainty is not carefully considered, wrong decisions will probably be made. Although many algorithms are used to classify determinate data, few classification algorithms have been proposed for uncertain data [4].

Extreme learning machine (ELM) is a simple and efficient learning algorithm for single-hidden layer feedforward neural networks (SLFNs) [13]. ELM-based uncertain data classification algorithms, such as AVG [5,19] based on expected values and SELM [8,18] based on sample points, have been proposed. However, three problems have not been addressed well in such ELM-based algorithms. (1) They model the data uncertainty with expected values or sample points, thus causing the loss of uncertain information. (2) They do not integrate the uncertain information into the ELM algorithm framework and thus can not deal with data uncertainty well. (3) Sample points need a large amount of computation, therefore the sample-based ELM methods are inefficient.

To solve the above problems, in this paper we propose a novel ELM-based uncertain data classification algorithm (UELM) to improve the existing ELM-based classification algorithms for uncertain data. Our main contributions are summarized as follows.

1. We model the data uncertainty by attribute intervals and probability density functions (PDFs), thus solving the problem of losing uncertain information in AVG and SELM.
2. We integrate the uncertain information into the ELM algorithm framework by modifying the received content in input layer and the hidden layer activation functions, which can deal with data uncertainty well.
3. Extensive experimental results show the superiority of our proposed algorithm UELM in terms of accuracy and efficiency.

2   Related Work

There has been a growing interest in uncertain data mining [4]. Uncertain data classification is an important component of uncertain data mining. In [1], density-based method is used for uncertain data classification. [7] studies how to classify uncertain data with support vector machine. In [19], an uncertain data classification algorithm UDT is proposed. UDT models the probability distribution information (uncertain information) with PDF and builds the tree with entropy. Naive Bayes classifiers [17], rule-based classifiers [14], nearest neighbour classifiers [5], artificial neural networks [11] and associative classification [15] are all extended to handle uncertain data. Except classification, uncertain data also have been extended into various traditional mining problems such as clustering [9,20], frequent pattern mining [10], outlier detection [3] and streams mining [2], etc.

Extreme learning machine (ELM) provides good generalization performance at extremely fast learning speed for learning the parameters of single-hidden layer feedforward neural networks (SLFNs) [13]. In [8,18], ELM-based uncertain data classification algorithm has been proposed. It models the data uncertainty with expected values and sample points, and modifies the prediction strategy. However, the loss of uncertain information and the inefficient problem exist in this solution. Thus, it can not deal with data uncertainty well. In this paper, our UELM algorithm takes full advantage of the uncertain information by modeling the data uncertainty with attribute intervals and probability density functions. Furthermore, we revise the input content and the hidden layer activation function of the ELM algorithm. And we greatly reduce the cost of the training and predicting time.

3   Preliminaries

In this section, we firstly introduce the way of modeling data uncertainty in UELM. Then, we give an overview of how ELM algorithm works.

3.1   Data Uncertainty Model

Generally, uncertain numerical attribute and uncertain categorical attribute are the most common attribute types encountered in uncertain data mining applications. In this paper, we focus on uncertain numerical attribute. Suppose that a training dataset contains n uncertain objects, $O = \{o_1, o_2, \ldots, o_n\}$ with d attributes, $A = \{A_1, A_2, \ldots, A_d\}$ and m class labels, $C = \{C_1, C_2, \ldots, C_m\}$. The i-th uncertain object $o_i \in O$ is represented by $V_i = \{v_{i,1}, v_{i,2}, \ldots, v_{i,d}\}$ with a class label $c_i \in C$. The j-th uncertain attribute value $v_{i,j}$ is a scalar random variable, thus $v_{i,j}$ is described not by a single value, but an attribute interval and a probability density function (PDF). And PDF is an useful tool to model the probability distribution information of uncertain objects. Suppose the value of random variable $v_{i,j}$, $x \in [l, r]$ and its PDF is denoted by $v_{i,j}.f(x)$, then,

$$\int_l^r v_{i,j}.f(x)\,dx = \begin{cases} 1, x \in [l, r] \\ 0, x \notin [l, r] \end{cases}. \tag{1}$$

Since most real applications involve random noise which follows Gaussian distribution [17,19], in this paper we assume that all the uncertain data obey Gaussian distribution.

3.2   Extreme Learning Machine

Extreme learning machine is a single-hidden layer feedforward network (SLFN) with an optimized learning algorithm [13]. All the hidden layer parameters are generated randomly without tuning. The output function of ELM is:

$$f_L(\boldsymbol{x}) = \sum_{i=1}^{L} \beta_i h_i(\boldsymbol{x}) = \boldsymbol{\beta}^T \boldsymbol{h}(\boldsymbol{x}), \tag{2}$$

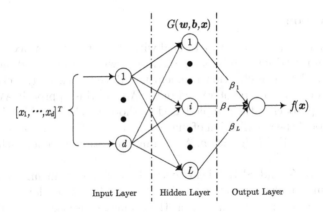

Fig. 1. ELM structure.

where $\boldsymbol{x} = [x_1, x_2, \ldots, x_d]^T$ is the input data, $\boldsymbol{\beta} = [\beta_1, \beta_2, \ldots, \beta_L]^T$ is the hidden-output layer weight vector and the $\boldsymbol{h}(\boldsymbol{x})$ is the output vector of the L hidden nodes. $\boldsymbol{h}(\boldsymbol{x})$ can be obtained by:

$$\boldsymbol{h}(\boldsymbol{x}) = G(\boldsymbol{w}, \boldsymbol{b}, \boldsymbol{x}) = G(\boldsymbol{w}^T\boldsymbol{x} + \boldsymbol{b}), \tag{3}$$

where $G(\boldsymbol{w}, \boldsymbol{b}, \boldsymbol{x})$ is a nonlinear function such as sigmoid function. $\boldsymbol{w}$ is the $d \times L$ weight matrix connecting the hidden nodes and the input nodes, and $\boldsymbol{b}$ is the bias vector of the hidden nodes, $\boldsymbol{b} = [b_1, b_2, \ldots, b_L]^T$. Figure 1 shows the ELM structure for binary classification and we can increase the number of output nodes for multi-classification. During the training process, $\boldsymbol{w}$ and $\boldsymbol{b}$ are generated randomly. The objective function of ELM is:

$$\min_{\beta} \| \boldsymbol{H}\boldsymbol{\beta} - \boldsymbol{T} \|, \tag{4}$$

where $\boldsymbol{H} = [\boldsymbol{h_1}(\boldsymbol{x_1})^T, \boldsymbol{h_2}(\boldsymbol{x_2})^T, \ldots, \boldsymbol{h_n}(\boldsymbol{x_n})^T]_{n \times L}^T$ is the hidden layer output matrix and $\boldsymbol{T} = [\boldsymbol{t_1^T}, \boldsymbol{t_2^T}, \ldots, \boldsymbol{t_n^T}]_{n \times m}^T$ are the class labels. m is the number of classes. With the least square method, the solution is:

$$\boldsymbol{\beta} = \boldsymbol{H}^\dagger \boldsymbol{T}, \tag{5}$$

where $\boldsymbol{H}^\dagger$ is called Moore-Penrose generalized inverse of matrix $\boldsymbol{H}$ [16]. And Formula (5) has the smallest norm of β among all the least square solutions. To handle uncertain data, we need to modify the activation function $G(\boldsymbol{w}, \boldsymbol{b}, \boldsymbol{x})$.

4   The Proposed Algorithm

In this section, we present our ELM-based uncertain data classification algorithm (UELM). We firstly analyse the insufficient of expected values and sample points. Then we model the data uncertainty with attribute intervals and PDFs. Furthermore, we modify the activation function of the hidden layer and the received content of input layer. Finally, we present the details of the UELM algorithm framework.

4.1   Motivation

Intuitively, a straightforward way to deal with the data uncertainty is to replace each uncertain attribute probability distribute with its expected value. Thus, the uncertain data classification problem is reduced back to the classification problem for determinate point-valued data. We call this approach AVG.

Another approach is the sample-based method, which is used in SELM. Sample points model the distribution of uncertain objects. Each sample point is classified to a class by ELM algorithm. According the voting method, each uncertain object predicts its class.

However, AVG and SELM lead to the loss of uncertain information more or less and may make a misclassification. Obviously, AVG adopts an expected point to represent an uncertain object, thus it may cause the loss of the distribute information of the uncertain object. In SELM, an uncertain object adopts many sample points to model the uncertain data. Although SELM takes more uncertain information into consideration than AVG, it is just an approximate representation of the uncertain object. Thus, SELM also loses a portion of uncertain information.

In UELM, attribute intervals and probability density functions (PDFs) are used to take full advantage of the uncertain information. The reason is that uncertain information represents the probability distribution information of uncertain data and PDF can deal with probability distribution information well. The class of an uncertain object will be assigned to the class which has the highest appearance probability calculated by attribute intervals and PDFs. Figure 2 shows the superiority of our proposed UELM algorithm against AVG and SELM in terms of uncertain data modeling.

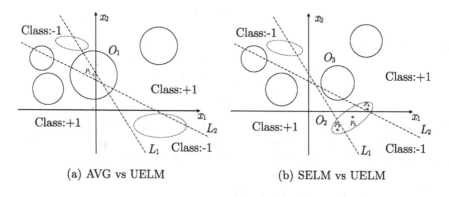

(a) AVG vs UELM   (b) SELM vs UELM

Fig. 2. Superiority of UELM

Figure 2 gives two examples of 2-dimensional uncertain data binary classification problem. Two linear classifiers L_1 and L_2 divide the whole data space into four pieces. Two small spaces stand for class -1 and the other two spaces represent class $+1$. The true class labels of the elliptical uncertain objects (dot line) are -1 and the circular uncertain objects (solid line) are $+1$. P_1 is the expected point of the uncertain object O_1. P_2, P_3 and P_4 are three sample points in the uncertain object O_2.

AVG vs UELM: As shown in Fig. 2(a), uncertain object O_1 lays in two different spaces of class $+1$ and class -1. P_1 represents its expected point. If we use AVG algorithm, O_1 will be assigned to class -1 because the expected point P_1 locates in the space of class -1. However, in UELM it is obvious that O_1 has a larger probability to be in the space of class $+1$ than in class -1. So the class of O_1 is $+1$.

SELM vs UELM: In Fig. 2(b), uncertain object O_2 has three sample points P_2, P_3 and P_4. Two sample points $P2$ and P_4 locate in the space of class $+1$ and only P_3 locates in the space of class -1. Therefore, if we use the SELM algorithm, according to the voting method, the class of uncertain object O_2 is class $+1$. Actually, O_2 belongs to class -1. Since UELM considers the full probability distribution information and predicts the class which has the highest appearance probability, UELM will perform the classification correctly.

According to the above analysis, AVG and SELM both lose the uncertain information more or less, and even worse, they may lead to a misclassification. So we choose attribute intervals and PDFs to model uncertain objects in UELM.

4.2 Modification of Activation Function

For ELM, it is hard to do anything different about the computing process of input layer and output layer. If we want to bring the uncertain information into ELM, the hidden layer is a good choice. Actually, each hidden layer node is a perceptron. Perceptron algorithm is as follows:

$$y = F(\sum_{i=1}^{d} w_i x_i + b), \quad F(x) = \begin{cases} 1, x \geqslant 0 \\ -1, x < 0 \end{cases}. \tag{6}$$

$F(x)$ is the activation function and y is the output of the perceptron. In order to deal with uncertain data, we need to modify the activation function. Taking uncertain object O_3 in Fig. 2(b) for an example, if L_2 is the perceptron, the criterion of O_3 belonging to class $+1$ is that more than half part of O_3 locates above L_2. As we can see, for classifier L_2 if the appearance probability of an uncertain object above L_2 is more than 0.5, its class label is $+1$, otherwise -1. We assume that $Prob(x \geqslant 0)$ denotes the probability of $x \geqslant 0$ and $z = \sum_{i=1}^{d} w_i x_i + b$. So we modify the $F(x)$ in Formula (6) to fit uncertain data as follows:

$$F(z) = \begin{cases} 1, Prob(z \geqslant 0) \geqslant 0.5 \\ -1, Prob(z \geqslant 0) < 0.5 \end{cases}. \tag{7}$$

According to the above discussion about the perceptron for uncertain data, the ELM algorithm can be changed with the modification of the activation function $G(\boldsymbol{w}, \boldsymbol{b}, \boldsymbol{x})$ as follows:

$$G(\boldsymbol{w}, \boldsymbol{b}, \boldsymbol{x}) = [g_1(\boldsymbol{w_1}, b_1, \boldsymbol{x}), \dots, g_i(\boldsymbol{w_i}, b_i, \boldsymbol{x}), \dots, g_L(\boldsymbol{w_L}, b_L, \boldsymbol{x})]^T,$$
$$g_i(\boldsymbol{w_i}, b_i, \boldsymbol{x}) = Prob(\boldsymbol{w_i}^T \boldsymbol{x} + b_i \geqslant 0), \tag{8}$$

where $\boldsymbol{w_i} = [w_{1i}, \ldots, w_{di}]^T$ and $\boldsymbol{b} = [b_1, b_2, \ldots, b_L]^T$. So the key point is how to compute $g_i(\boldsymbol{w_i}, b_i, \boldsymbol{x})$.

We assume that the distribution of uncertain data obeys Gaussian distribution and $x_i \sim N(\mu_i, \sigma_i^2)$. As mentioned earlier, $z_i = \boldsymbol{w_i^T x} + b_i$. Suppose that each attribute is independent of the others, so z_i will have a Gaussian distribution as:

$$z_i \sim N(\boldsymbol{w_i^T \mu} + b_i, (diag(\boldsymbol{w_i})\boldsymbol{w_i})^T (diag(\boldsymbol{\sigma})\boldsymbol{\sigma})), \tag{9}$$

where $diag(\boldsymbol{w_i})$ represents a square diagonal matrix with the elements of vector $\boldsymbol{w_i}$ on the main diagonal and $\boldsymbol{\mu} = [\mu_1, \mu_2, \ldots, \mu_d]^T$, $\boldsymbol{\sigma} = [\sigma_1, \sigma_2, \ldots, \sigma_d]^T$. In our UELM algorithm, uncertain data can be expressed by probability density function. Therefore, based on Formula (8), we get:

$$g_i(z_i) = Prob(z_i \geqslant 0) = \int_0^{+\infty} f(z_i)\,dz_i, \tag{10}$$

where $f(z_i)$ denotes the PDF of z_i and $g_i(z_i) = g_i(\boldsymbol{w_i}, b_i, \boldsymbol{x})$. z_i obeys Gaussian distribution, so we can get $g_i(z_i)$ as:

$$g_i(z_i) = \int_0^{+\infty} \frac{1}{\sqrt{2\pi}\sigma_{z_i}} exp(-\frac{(z_i - \mu_{z_i})^2}{2\sigma_{z_i}^2})\,dz_i, \tag{11}$$

where μ_{z_i} represents the expected value of z_i and σ_{z_i} represents the standard deviation of z_i as defined in Formula (9). Formula (11) shows the computing method of the probability over $[0, +\infty)$ of uncertain object $\boldsymbol{x}$. However, the premise of Formula (11) is that the area coverage of uncertain object $\boldsymbol{x}$ is $(-\infty, +\infty)$. Actually, each attribute of the uncertain object $\boldsymbol{x}$ has an interval and $z_i = \boldsymbol{w_i^T x} + b_i$. Thus, the interval of z_i can be calculated by the attribute intervals of uncertain object $\boldsymbol{x}$ and parameters $(\boldsymbol{w_i}, b_i)$. Suppose the interval of z_i is $[a_{z_i}, b_{z_i}]$ and $[c_{z_i}, d_{z_i}]$ is the intersection of $[a_{z_i}, b_{z_i}]$ and $[0, +\infty)$, so the probability of z_i over $[0, +\infty)$ is:

$$g_i(z_i) = \frac{\int_{c_{z_i}}^{d_{z_i}} \frac{1}{\sqrt{2\pi}\sigma_{z_i}} exp(-\frac{(z_i - \mu_{z_i})^2}{2\sigma_{z_i}^2})\,dz_i}{\int_{a_{z_i}}^{b_{z_i}} \frac{1}{\sqrt{2\pi}\sigma_{z_i}} exp(-\frac{(z_i - \mu_{z_i})^2}{2\sigma_{z_i}^2})\,dz_i}. \tag{12}$$

And then, $G(\boldsymbol{w}, \boldsymbol{b}, \boldsymbol{x})$ can be obtained based on Formula (12). In Sect. 3.2, $h(\boldsymbol{x}) = G(\boldsymbol{w}, \boldsymbol{b}, \boldsymbol{x})$ and $\boldsymbol{H} = [h_1(\boldsymbol{x_1})^T, h_2(\boldsymbol{x_2})^T, \ldots, h_n(\boldsymbol{x_n})^T]_{n \times L}^T$, thus we get $\boldsymbol{H}$. During the computation process, UELM needs the expected values and standard deviations of uncertain data, so the input layer in Fig. 1 is revised to receive $(\boldsymbol{\mu}, \boldsymbol{\sigma})$ rather than $\boldsymbol{x}$.

4.3   Algorithm Framework

The algorithm framework of UELM consists of three parts: initialization process, training process and predicting process, which are shown in Algorithm 1.

Algorithm 1. UELM Algorithm

Input:

D_{train}: training dataset; D_{test}: testing dataset; L: the number of hidden nodes;

Output:

C_{test}: prediction of class labels;

1: // Initialization process
2: Generate parameters w and b randomly;
3: // Training process
4: Calculate the interval of z_i based on $z_i = w_i^T x + b_i$;
5: Calculate the intersection of $[0, +\infty)$ and the interval of z_i which is obtained by step 4;
6: Calculate the distribution parameters $(\mu_{z_i}, \sigma_{z_i})$ based on Formula (9);
7: Calculate H_{train} based on $H = [h_1(x_1)^T, h_2(x_2)^T, \ldots, h_n(x_n)^T]_{n \times L}^T$, $h(x) = G(w, b, x)$ and Formula (12);
8: Calculate the weight β based on Formula (5);
9: // Predicting process
10: Calculate H_{test} with D_{test}, w and b, according to step 4, 5, 6 and 7;
11: Calculate the class label for each uncertain object in D_{test} with β and H_{test} based on Formula (2).
12: Return C_{test};

Initialization Process: Firstly, we mine the uncertain information from uncertain dataset such as attribute intervals and the distribution parameters (μ and σ if it is Gaussian distribution). And then, we generate parameters w and b randomly and assign the number of hidden nodes with L.

Training Process: With the uncertain information of training dataset, the interval of z_i and the distribution parameters $(\mu_{z_i}, \sigma_{z_i})$ can be obtained based on Formula (9). And then, we calculate $g_i(z_i)$ based on Formula (12). According to Formula (8), we can obtain $G(w, b, x)$. In Sect. 3.2, we know that $h(x) = G(w, b, x)$ and $H = [h_1(x_1)^T, h_2(x_2)^T, \ldots, h_n(x_n)^T]_{n \times L}^T$. Thus, we will get H_{train}. Finally, the weight matrix β will be obtained based on Formula (5).

Predicting Process: As well as the training process, we get the H_{test} with the testing dataset D_{test}. With H_{test} and β which is obtained in training process, each test uncertain object will get m values based on Formula (2). m is the number of classes. Finally, the class which has the maximum value will be assigned to the class of the test uncertain object.

5   Experiments

In this section, we present the experimental results of expected value-based algorithm (AVG), sample-based ELM algorithm (SELM) and our proposed algorithm UELM on six real datasets (see Table 1) taken from the UCI Machine Learning Repository [6]. All the experiments are implemented with Matlab R2015a and executed on a computer with an Intel Core i5 3.2 GHz processor and 16GB RAM.

Table 1. Datasets

Datasets	Training tuples	No. of features	No. of classes	Test tuples
Blood transfusion	748	4	2	5-fold
Breast cancer	569	30	2	5-fold
Glass	214	9	6	5-fold
Page blocks	5473	10	5	5-fold
Satellite	4435	36	6	2000
Japanese vowel	270	12	9	370

5.1   Datasets and Settings

For the purpose of our experiments, these six datasets contain mostly numerical attributes. There are two kinds of datasets: the dataset without data uncertainty (expect "Japanese Vowel") and the dataset with data uncertainty ("Japanese Vowel"). Among the six datasets, "Satellite" and "Japanese Vowel" are already divided into training and testing tuples. For the other four datasets, we use 5-fold cross validation to measure the accuracy and time efficiency. Table 1 shows the details of the datasets.

Due to a lack of real uncertain datasets, except "Japanese Vowel", we have inserted the uncertain information into the selected datasets, following [5,19]. The modeling process of uncertain information is determined as follows: Suppose A_j^{min} and A_j^{max} are the minimum and maximum values of attribute A_j respectively. For each object o_i and for each attribute A_j, the uncertain attribute value $v_{i,j}$ has the uncertain interval $[v_{i,j} - (v_{i,j} - A_j^{min}) * U * rand1, v_{i,j} + (A_j^{max} - v_{i,j}) * U * rand2]$, where U controls the uncertainty degree of uncertain data. $rand1$ and $rand2$ denote the random numbers in the interval of $[0, 1]$.

For AVG and SELM, we need to generate sample points. Suppose $[a_{i,j}, b_{i,j}]$ is the uncertain attribute interval which is generated above. And then, $a_{i,j} + (b_{i,j} - a_{i,j}) * rand3$ is a sample point, where $rand3$ is a normally distributed random number in the interval of $[0, 1]$. For the AVG algorithm, the input data for the ELM algorithm use the expected values of the generated sample points above. For the SELM algorithm, the input data are the generated sample points above.

For our UELM algorithm, each uncertain object o_i use the original value $v_{i,j}$ as the mean value $\mu_{i,j}$ for each uncertain attribute A_j. And $\sigma_{i,j} = 0.25 * (v_{max}^j - v_{min}^j) * U$.

Each value in $\boldsymbol{w}$ of ELM randomly generates in the interval of $[-1, 1]$ and each value in $\boldsymbol{b}$ of ELM randomly generates in the interval of $[0, 1]$. We vary the uncertainty degree U to be 0.01, 0.05, 0.1, 0.2. For AVG and SELM algorithm, the number of sample points is 100 [5,17,19]. Another user-specified parameter is the number of the hidden nodes L. In our experiments, L has six candidate values 50, 100, 300, 500, 800, 1000. Each dataset has a fixed L, and with the fixed L three algorithms all achieve the best accuracy over different L settings.

5.2 Accuracy

Table 2 shows the accuracy results of applying AVG, SELM and UELM to the six datasets. To better show the best potential improvement, for each dataset the results in bold represent the highest accuracy among the three algorithms with the same uncertainty degree. From the table, we see that our proposed UELM algorithm always achieves higher accuracy than AVG and SELM. For example, UELM improves the classification accuracy by about 10% for the "Satellite" dataset. The reason is that the computation of expected values or sample points may cause the loss of uncertain information and without uncertain information the ELM algorithm framework can not deal with uncertain data well. This confirms our hypothesis that more accurate classifier can be learnt by considering the uncertain information with attribute intervals and PDFs rather than the expected values or sample points and integrating the uncertain information into the ELM algorithm framework. All in all, UELM always gives better accuracies for different algorithms over a wide range of uncertainty degree.

Table 2. Accuracy results

Datasets	Methods	Uncertainty degree			
		1%	5%	10%	20%
Blood transfusion	AVG	75.98%	76.25%	77.95%	75.98%
	SELM	76.21%	76.21%	75.95%	77.02%
	UELM	**81.15%**	**79.16%**	**80.08%**	**81.67%**
Breast Cancer	AVG	91.41%	88.21%	91.92%	93.16%
	SELM	96.67%	97.20%	97.72%	98.08%
	UELM	**97.56%**	**98.24%**	**98.59%**	**99.65%**
Glass	AVG	61.30%	61.30%	61.61%	67.20%
	SELM	67.29%	65.86%	66.94%	73.83%
	UELM	**72.73%**	**77.64%**	**72.05%**	**78.94%**
Page blocks	AVG	96.07%	95.63%	94.79%	93.62%
	SELM	95.93%	94.65%	94.30%	93.20%
	UELM	**96.40%**	**96.46%**	**96.47%**	**96.51%**
Satellite	AVG	78.50%	79.15%	78.70%	77.90%
	SELM	78.75%	79.70%	78.85%	80.95%
	UELM	**88.85%**	**88.95%**	**89.35%**	**90.20%**
Japanese vowel	AVG	94.86%			
	SELM	96.76%			
	UELM	**97.57%**			

5.3 Efficiency

Figure 3 shows the training and test time comparison on different datasets. The horizontal axis represents the uncertainty degree U. The vertical axis, which is in log scale, represents the execution time in seconds. For dataset "Japanese Vowel", since its data uncertainty is taken from raw data, the horizontal axis of Fig. 3(f) doesn't represent uncertainty degree.

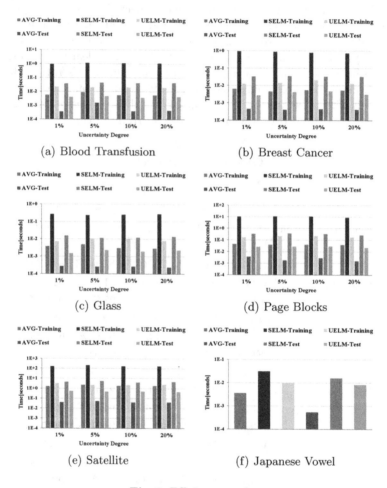

Fig. 3. Efficiency results

As the efficiency results shown, UELM performs better than SELM in both the training time and the test time, but not better than AVG due to the integral computation in UELM. For example, "Satellite" dataset takes 153 s during the training process with SELM, however, UELM only takes 3 s. In the sample-based ELM algorithm SELM, the computation of large number of sample points leads to a sharp drop in time efficiency. Our UELM algorithm is more effective than SELM by modeling the data uncertainty with attribute intervals and PDFs, and redesigning the ELM algorithm framework. All in all, our UELM algorithm is competitive compared to other algorithms in terms of efficiency.

6   Conclusions and Future Work

In this paper, we proposed a novel ELM-based uncertain data classification algorithm UELM. The proposed algorithm can efficiently solve the remaining problems of the existing ELM-based methods by modeling uncertain data with exact probability density function (PDF) and redesigning the traditional ELM algorithm framework. Experimental results showed the superiority of our UELM algorithm in terms of accuracy and efficiency. For future work, we will extend the method to multi-layer neural networks with connecting many ELMs together and we will integrate the statistic feature extraction methods into ELM such as PCA, GMM, restricted Boltzmann machines.

References

1. Aggarwal, C.C.: On density based transforms for uncertain data mining. In: Proceedings of ICDE, pp. 866–875. IEEE (2007)
2. Aggarwal, C.C.: On high dimensional projected clustering of uncertain data streams. In: Proceedings of ICDE, pp. 1152–1154. IEEE (2009)
3. Aggarwal, C.C., Philip, S.Y.: Outlier detection with uncertain data. In: SDM, vol. 8, pp. 483–493. SIAM (2008)
4. Aggarwal, C.C., Yu, P.S.: A survey of uncertain data algorithms and applications. IEEE Trans. Knowl. Data Eng. **21**(5), 609–623 (2009)
5. Angiulli, F., Fassetti, F.: Nearest neighbor-based classification of uncertain data. ACM Trans. Knowl. Disc. Data **7**(1), 1–34 (2013)
6. Asuncion, A., Newman, D.: UCI machine learning repository (2007)
7. Bi, J., Zhang, T.: Support vector classification with input data uncertainty. In: Proceedings of NIPS, pp. 161–168 (2004)
8. Cao, K., Wang, G., Han, D., Bai, M., Li, S.: An algorithm for classification over uncertain data based on extreme learning machine. Neurocomputing **174**, 194–202 (2016)
9. Cormode, G., Mcgregor, A.: Approximation algorithms for clustering uncertain data. In: Proceedings of PODS, pp. 191–200 (2008)
10. Gao, C., Wang, J.: Direct mining of discriminative patterns for classifying uncertain data. In: Proceedings of SIGKDD, pp. 861–870 (2010)
11. Ge, J., Xia, Y., Nadungodage, C.: UNN: a neural network for uncertain data classification. In: Zaki, M.J., Yu, J.X., Ravindran, B., Pudi, V. (eds.) PAKDD 2010. LNCS (LNAI), vol. 6118, pp. 449–460. Springer, Heidelberg (2010). doi:10.1007/978-3-642-13657-3_48
12. Han, J., Pei, J., Kamber, M.: Data Mining: Concepts and Techniques. Elsevier, New York (2011)
13. Huang, G.B., Zhu, Q.Y., Siew, C.K.: Extreme learning machine: theory and applications. Neurocomputing **70**(1), 489–501 (2006)

14. Qin, B., Xia, Y., Prabhakar, S., Tu, Y.: A rule-based classification algorithm for uncertain data. In: Proceedings of ICDE, pp. 1633–1640. IEEE (2009)
15. Qin, X., Zhang, Y., Li, X., Wang, Y.: Associative classifier for uncertain data. In: Chen, L., Tang, C., Yang, J., Gao, Y. (eds.) WAIM 2010. LNCS, vol. 6184, pp. 692–703. Springer, Heidelberg (2010). doi:10.1007/978-3-642-14246-8_66
16. Rao, C.R., Mitra, S.K.: Generalized Inverse of Matrices and Its Applications, vol. 7. Wiley, New York (1971)
17. Ren, J., Lee, S.D., Chen, X., Kao, B., Cheng, R., Cheung, D.: Naive bayes classification of uncertain data. In: Proceedings of ICDM, pp. 944–949. IEEE (2009)
18. Sun, Y., Yuan, Y., Wang, G.: Extreme learning machine for classification over uncertain data. Neurocomputing **128**, 500–506 (2014)
19. Tsang, S., Kao, B., Yip, K.Y., Ho, W.S., Lee, S.D.: Decision trees for uncertain data. IEEE Trans. Knowl. Data Eng. **23**(1), 64–78 (2011)
20. Zhang, X., Liu, H., Zhang, X., Liu, X.: Novel density-based clustering algorithms for uncertain data. In: Proceedings of AAAI, pp. 2191–2197 (2014)

SPGLAD: A Self-paced Learning-Based Crowdsourcing Classification Model

Xianchao Zhang[1], Heng Shi[1], Yuangang Li[2,3], and Wenxin Liang[1]([✉])

[1] School of Software Technology, Dalian University of Technology,
Dalian 116024, China
{xczhang,wxliang}@dlut.edu.cn, shiheng@mail.dlut.edu.cn
[2] Shanghai University of Finance and Economics, Shanghai 200433, China
[3] Goldpac Limited, Zhuhai 519070, China
gary.li@goldpac.com

Abstract. Crowdsourcing platforms like Amazon's Mechanical Turk provide fast and effective solutions of collecting massive datasets for performing tasks in domains such as image classification, information retrieval, etc. Crowdsourcing quality control plays an essential role in such systems. However, existing algorithms are prone to get stuck in a bad local optimum because of ill-defined datasets. To overcome the above drawbacks, we propose a novel self-paced quality control model integrating a priority-based sample-picking strategy. The proposed model ensures the evident samples do better efforts during iterations. We also empirically demonstrate that the proposed self-paced learning strategy promotes common quality control methods.

Keywords: Crowdsourcing · Self-paced learning · Quality control

1 Introduction

Crowdsourcing becomes increasingly popular in recent years, with the belief that the wisdom of the crowd is superior to the judgements of individuals. Crowdsourcing platforms, such as Amazon Mechanical Turk[1] and CrowdFlower[2], distribute tasks to workers that are paid for their answers. Achieving domain knowledge by crowdsourcing is more convenient and cheaper than engaging experts.

It is an important problem of crowdsourcing to extract the truth from multiple workers' answers. Crowdsourcing quality control methods aggregate answers provided by conflictual data sources. Particularly, crowdsourcing quality control methods are applied in classification tasks, in which workers are requested to classify objects to corresponding categories. There are several classical classification tasks in crowdsourcing such as indicating whether a photo contains people

---

This work was supported by 863 project of China (No. 2015AA015403) and NSFC (No. 61632019).

[1] http://www.mturk.com.
[2] http://crowdflower.com.

© Springer International Publishing AG 2017
U Kang et al. (Eds.): PAKDD 2017 Workshops, LNAI 10526, pp. 189–201, 2017.
DOI: 10.1007/978-3-319-67274-8_17

or not, judging whether URLs and queries are relevant or not and ranking web pages. Majority voting (MV) is a direct solution to this problem in a heuristic way. However, MV fails to take into account the reliabilities of different workers and difficulties of objects. To overcome this problem, Whitehill et al. [11] proposes the Generative model of Labels Abilities and Difficulties (GLAD) model which emphasizes the differences of workers and objects.

However, crowdsourcing data in real-world is often sparse and imbalanced with different workers and objects. The reliabilities of workers who contribute lots of data samples are easy to learn. Nevertheless, it's difficult for models to evaluate workers providing fewer samples. Evaluating the difficulty of objects also has the same problem. Most of probabilistic models treat samples with the same priority during optimization, which carry negative impacts to following iterations. Self-paced learning [6] formulates the learning problem as a concise biconvex problem and guides the learning process according to the easiness of samples. In self-paced learning, data samples with different difficulties are learnt in different paces, which avoids the drawbacks in traditional crowdsourcing models and achieves better classification results.

In this paper, we propose a novel self-paced probabilistic model named Self-Paced GLAD (SPGLAD). The proposed model integrates a priority-based sample-picking strategy with GLAD model to determine easy samples that are learnt firstly. SPGLAD also provide a method to get proper a priori for self-paced parameters. Consequently, SPGLAD smoothly guides the learning process to emphasize the patterns of reliable samples rather than those of noisy and confusing ones and obtains the learning robustness.

We formulate the proposed model as a fully corrective optimization in crowdsourcing. The contributions of this paper are summarized as follows:

1. We propose a self-paced crowdsourcing algorithm (SPGLAD) which dynamically incorporates samples into learning from easy ones to difficult ones. We also define the conception easiness of crowdsourcing data samples and propose a method to get proper prior distributions of parameters.
2. We explain SPGLAD as a probabilistic graph model and illustrate that our model is an effective approximation of generative models.
3. We empirically show that SPGLAD outperforms other models without a self-paced process on both synthetic and real-world datasets.

The paper is structured as follows. Section 2 reviews related work. Section 3 introduces the preliminary notation and the GLAD model. Section 4 details SPGLAD models and its probabilistic inference. Section 5 presents our experimental settings and the empirical evaluation of our method on real-world datasets. Section 6 concludes the paper and presents directions for future work.

2   Related Work

2.1   Crowdsourcing

Aggregating crowdsourcing data attracts a lot of research efforts, and yields many insightful discoveries. An advanced approach for label aggregation is suggested by Dawid and Skene [2]. They assume that each worker has a latent confusion matrix for labeling and performs equally well across all items in a common class. To solve the difference of objects in the same class, Zhou [14,15] proposes a minimax entropy principle for crowdsourcing. Yin [13] proposes an iterative truth finder algorithm by simultaneously accessing the trustworthiness of each source. Venanzi [9] gave a community-based Bayesian models, which assume workers in the same group share the similar confuse matrix.

Recently, some researchers introduced active or adaptive learning methods [3,5] into crowdsourcing to improve accuracy with less labels. They focus on selecting workers or objects during task distributions, and reducing budget with better results. But those methods assumed a long-term labeling process for workers which is hard to guarantee for general crowdsourcing platform. Other methods [7,10] are also proposed by taking full advantage of text and multi-media data to use more information in special crowdsourcing data.

2.2   Self-paced Learning

The self-paced learning is inspired by the learning process of human that gradually incorporates the training samples into learning samples from easy ones to complex ones. Different from curriculum learning [1] which learns the data in a predefined order based on prior knowledge, self-paced learning choose samples dynamically. Self-paced learning is applied in many different domains, such as image classification [6] and matrix factorization [12].

In this paper, we propose the definition of easiness in crowdsourcing and introduces self-paced learning into GLAD model. Besides, we also give a priori like curriculum learning based on domain knowledge in crowdsourcing which helps the self-paced learning process during cold start.

3   Preliminaries

3.1   Notations

Considering that $W \geq 1$ workers label $N \geq 1$ objects. Each of objects has $C \geq 2$ categories to choose from. While, exactly one of the C categories is correct. Let l_{ij} be the category which i-th worker chooses for j-th object. z_j is the correct category of j-th object. The ability of i-th worker is modeled by $\alpha_i \in (-\infty, +\infty)$, workers with higher abilities will give more correct labels. Workers with negative α_i are considered as spammer. For objects, we use the parameter $1/\beta_j \in (0, +\infty)$ to model the difficulty of labeling j-th object. Objects with $\beta_j \to +\infty$ means this label task is easy, hence most of workers can do it correctly.

Since we assume labeling task is assigned to workers randomly, both the number of data samples each worker given and the times of each object been labeled is different. c_j is the number of times that j-th object has been labeled. t_i is the number of labels that i-th worker has given. In general, for a given dataset $\mathcal{D} = \{l_{1,1}, l_{1,2}, ..., l_{W,N}\}$, crowdsourcing quality control algorithm should estimate the ability of workers $\{\alpha_i\}$, the difficulty of objects $\{1/\beta_j\}$ and give the correct categories $\{z_j\}$.

3.2 GLAD

Whitehill et al. [11] proposed a generative probabilistic model named GLAD which has been successfully applied to crowdsourcing problems in previous works. They make an assumption that labels given by the i-th worker to the j-th object are generated by Eq. (1).

$$p(l_{ij} = z_j | \alpha_i, \beta_j) = \frac{1}{1 + e^{-\alpha_i \beta_j}}. \tag{1}$$

Under this assumption, parameters of the GLAD model can be estimated through Expectation-Maximization (EM) approach to get a maximum likelihood estimator, where margined likelihood is shown in Eq. (2).

$$p(L | \alpha, \beta, \theta, \nu, \mu, \sigma, \pi) =$$

$$\prod_{i=1}^{W} p(\alpha_i | \theta_i, \nu_i) \prod_{j}^{N} p(\beta_j | \mu_j, \sigma_j) \prod_{l_{ij} \in L} (\sum_{z \in C} p(l_{ij} | z_j, \alpha_i, \beta_j) p(z_j)). \tag{2}$$

The GLAD model can also be used with an explicit prior over each α_i, β_j and z_j. For example, the workers with bad behaviors before may get a prior with low mean and high variance and the objects which workers often get confused with tend to be generated from a norm with higher mean.

3.3 Limitation of GLAD

Two problems need to be solved when we use the GLAD model in real world datasets. First, because of non-convexity of object functions, the GLAD model often get stuck into bad local minima.

Second, the GLAD model treats all data samples with the same priority. Table 1 shows a toy dataset from AdultContent dataset. There are also other labels given by worker1, but worker2 only give 2 labels. Since worker2 is one of few workers who gives labels for url3 and give the correct answer for url1, worker2 is tend to be considered with higher ability than worker1 who give lots of examples. In fact, worker2 is a common worker or even a spammer. It is hard for models to estimate the ability with a small number of samples contributed by worker2 at the beginning of optimization.

Some methods [8,11] are proposed to solve this problem, such as adding prior distributions or asking users to provide other information from workers. Those methods need more prior knowledge and hard to implement since we can't assume workers always give objective and truthful information.

4 Self-paced GLAD

The basic idea of the proposed model is to introduce self-paced learning to the crowdsourcing algorithm. Our self-paced learning model relieves itself from lack of a readily computable easiness measure for samples. In the context of labeling

Table 1. AdultContent DataSet and ground truth

Worker	Website	Category		Website	Truth
worker1	url1	1		url1	1
worker2	url1	1		url2	0
worker1	url2	1		url3	0
worker1	url3	1		...	...
...	...	...			

process with a latent variable z, we introduce a parameter w to representing the easiness of samples.

We define the easiness in two ways:

- **Assumption I.** A sample is easy if the label can be generated with a high probability by the proposed model.
- **Assumption II.** A sample is easy if we have enough data to predict workers' ability and the true labels of objects.

These two assumptions are somewhat related: If we get enough data to predict workers' ability or objects' categories, those are more likely to be generated by the model with higher probability. **Assumption II** is the precondition for estimating easiness in **Assumption I**, which should be handled with prior knowledge acquired from the dataset. Moreover, easiness in **Assumption I** is dynamic and should be estimated in each iteration.

In order to handle those two assumptions, we build up a novel iterative self-paced quality control algorithm. The algorithm guide the learning from difficult samples to easy ones in a self-paced way.

4.1   Model Overview

In the above argument, we assumed a given **w** for each sample. However, in order to operationalize self-paced learning, we need a strategy for simultaneously choosing the easy samples and learning the parameter w during each iteration. To this end, we add **w** to the generate model and give a prior to it. For each label, we use a w_{ij} to handle **Assumption I** and optimize Eq. (3).

$$\mathbf{w}_{t+1} = \operatorname*{argmax}_{w \in R^d} \Big(r(w) + L(\alpha, \beta, l, w) \Big), \tag{3}$$

where $r(.)$ is a regularization function which we is discussed later and $L(.)$ is log-likelihood for EM. We now modify the above optimization problem by introducing binary variables $v_{ij} \in \{0, 1\}$ that indicate whether the i-th sample is easy or not according to Eq. (4). Only easy samples contribute to the objective function.

$$(\mathbf{w}_{t+1}, \mathbf{v}_{t+1}) = \operatorname*{argmax}_{w \in R^d} \Big(r(w) + L(\alpha, \beta, l, v) \Big). \tag{4}$$

For the prior distribution part, we hope prior can handle **Assumption II**. This means prior distribution should use c_j and t_i for parameters. Moreover, v_{ij} can be seen as a binary variable following binomial distribution with parameter w_{ij}. Thus, we naturally chose beta distribution as priori. Considering these two parts, we use Eq. (5) to generate the prior distribution of w_{ij}

$$w_{ij} \sim Beta(c_j * t_i, \lambda(W * N)). \tag{5}$$

In real datasets, we find that $W * N \gg c_j * t_i$. Hence, we use λ as a super parameter to control the strength of prior by letting $\frac{c_j * t_i}{\lambda(W * N)}$ be proper value for datasets.

4.2 Parameter Estimation

Since our model involves unobserved latent variables and the object function is difficult to optimize, we use the Expectation Maximization (EM) algorithm to estimate them. Parameters is updated separately in three steps as followings.

In the **E-Step**, z_{jc} stands for that the true category of j-th object is c. Then, we compute the posterior probabilities of all $z_{jc} \in C$ as

$$p(z_{jc}|l, \alpha, \beta, v) = \frac{p(z_{jc}) \prod_i v_{ij} p(l_{ij}|z_{jc}, \alpha_i, \beta_j)}{\sum_{c' \in C} p(z_{jc'} \prod_i v_{ij} p(l_{ij}|z_{jc'}, \alpha_i, \beta_j))}, \tag{6}$$

Since not each worker give labels for each object, we use $v_{ij} = 0$ for the i-th workers who don't labeled the j-th object.

In the **M-Step**, the goal is to maximize $Q(\alpha, \beta)$ as

$$Q(\alpha, \beta) = E[\ln p(l, z|\alpha, \beta, v)]$$
$$E\left[\ln \prod_j \prod_c \left(p(z_{jc}) \prod_i v_{ij} p(l_{ij}|\alpha_i, \beta_j, z_{jc})\right)\right] \tag{7}$$

This Q is maximized by gradient ascending respect to the parameters α and β. We define p^c as

$$p^c = p(l_{ij}|z_{jc}, \alpha_i, \beta_j) = \begin{cases} \frac{1}{1+e^{-\alpha_i\beta_j}} & l_{ij} = z_{jc} \\ \frac{1}{C-1}\left(\frac{e^{-\alpha_i\beta_j}}{1+e^{-\alpha_i\beta_j}}\right) & l_{ij} \neq z_{jc} \end{cases} \tag{8}$$

Then, we update α and β as following

$$\frac{\partial Q}{\partial \alpha} = \sum_j \sum_c p^c[v_{ij}\delta(l_{ij}, z_{jc})\beta_j], \tag{9}$$

$$\frac{\partial Q}{\partial \beta} = \sum_i \sum_c p^c[v_{ij}\delta(l_{ij}, z_{jc})\alpha_i], \tag{10}$$

where $\delta(a, b)$ is the Kronecker delta function. $\delta(a, b)$ is 1 if the variables are equal, and 0 otherwise.

Algorithm 1. Self-paced GLAD

1: Random initialize the parameters $\alpha = (\alpha_i)_{i=1}^{W}$ and $\beta = (\beta_j)_{j=1}^{N}$ respectively.
2: $n \leftarrow 0$
3: **repeat**
4:    **E-step:**
5:    Compute $p(z_{jc}|l, \alpha, \beta, v)$ as in Eq. (6)
6:    **M-step:**
7:    Update α as in Eq. (9) with v^n
8:    Update β_{n+1} as in Eq. (10) with v^n
9:    **Update V:**
10:   **repeat**
11:      Compute w^{n+1} as in Eq. (11).
12:      Compute v^{n+1} as in Eq. (12).
13:   **until** convergence or maxiter
14:   decrease ξ
15:   $n \leftarrow n + 1$
16: **until** convergence or maxiter

Updating W and V is described in Sect. 4.1, w_{ij} is calculated following Eq. (11).

$$w_{ij} = \sum_c p(z_{jc})p(l_{ij}|z_{jc}, \alpha_i, \beta_j) + p(w_{ij}). \tag{11}$$

The first part of Eq. (11) measures the easiness of l_{ij} by probability of generating l_{ij} with parameters during iterations. $p(w_{ij})$ is the prior distribution of w_{ij} from Eq. (5).

Then, v_{ij} is

$$v_{ij} = \begin{cases} 1 & if \ w_{ij} \geq \xi \\ 0 & if \ w_{ij} < \xi \end{cases}. \tag{12}$$

Taking ξ as the threshold to control the pace at which the model learns new examples, and it is usually iteratively decreased during optimization.

At the beginning of iterations, the first part of Eq. (11) tends to be small. The $p(w_{ij})$ helps model to choose samples from a prior view. After the model have learned data well, the first part of Eq. (11) is large enough and the model uses it to choose easy samples. With ξ decreasing, almost all samples is chosen. The pseudo-code of the Self-Paced GLAD algorithm is shown in Algorithm (1).

4.3 Relation with Graph Model

It's easy to find the relation between the self-paced model and the traditional generative graph model. The easiness of samples which plays an important role in self-paced learning can been considered as a kind of regularizer. But w is calculated with the whole model instead of some parameters. Here, for w and

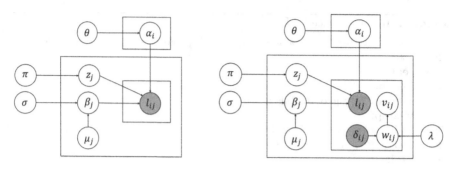

Fig. 1. GLAD   **Fig. 2.** Self-paced GLAD

v in self-paced GLAD model, it is considered as latent variables generated from domain specific attributes.

The graphs of GLAD and SPGLAD model are shown in Figs. 1 and 2 respectively. Log likelihood of posterior distribution is shown in Eq. 13.

$$\Theta = \ln P(L|\theta, \pi, \sigma, \lambda) =$$
$$\sum_i p(\alpha_i) + \sum_j p(\beta_j) + \sum_{ij} v_{ij} \ln \left(\sum_c p(l_{ij}|z_{jc}, \alpha_i, \beta_j) \right) \tag{13}$$
$$+ \sum_{ij} \left(p(v_{ij}|w_{ij}) + p(w_{ij}|\sigma, \lambda) \right).$$

To update v_{ij} we need to calculate Eq. (14).

$$\frac{\partial \Theta}{\partial v_{ij}} = \ln \left(\sum_c p(l_{ij}|z_{jc}, \alpha_i, \beta_j) \right) + r(w_{ij}). \tag{14}$$

Comparing Eqs. 11 and 14, we find our method is approximate solution for this generative model. But our way in getting w_{ij} and v_{ij} is more efficient since we calculate w_{ij} with ξ directly instead of using optimization methods.

4.4   Complexity Analysis

In each E-step of our model, it takes $\mathcal{O}(WNC)$ operations to compute for each $p(z_{jc}|l, \alpha, \beta, v)$ since we need to go through every sample and category for object j. In each M-step, we compute α with $\mathcal{O}(WCT)$ operations and β with $\mathcal{O}(NCT)$ operations which T is the number of maximal iterations in the gradient ascending method. At last, we need $\mathcal{O}(WN)$ operations to get w_{ij} and v_{ij}. Thus, our model has a time complexity of $\mathcal{O}(M(WNC + WCT + WN))$, where M is the number of iterations.

5   Experiments

In this section, we compare the proposed Self-Paced GLAD model with other crowdsourcing quality control algorithms in both synthetic dataset and real-world datasets. The baseline algorithms are as follows.

- **Majority Voting (MV):** The MV method estimates the aggregated label as the one with the most votes, where each vote is considered with equal weight.
- **Dawid & Skene (D&S)** [2]: The D&S model allows the joint estimation of the items' true labels and the workers' confusion matrices.
- **3-Estimates** [4]: Galland proposed a probabilistic model to estimate source reliability.
- **GLAD** [11]: The GLAD model takes difference of workers and objects into account, and take truth label as latent variables.

We further compare two variants of our model to show the benefit of adding prior for w. SPGLAD-a is a variant of our SPGLAD model without setting prior for easiness of samples. Comparison with these two baselines can show that objects with few labels and workers given few labels cause our model get stuck in local optimum at the beginning of iterations.

5.1   Performance Metric

To evaluate the performance of each method, *Error Rate* is used as evaluation metric, which is defined as the number of incorrectly labeled objects divided by the total number of objects N. A lower error rate means that the method's estimations is closer the ground truth, and the method is better than those with higher error rates.

5.2   Synthetic Datasets

Following Whitehill et al. [11], we explore the performance of our model using dataset generated by ourselves in two-category problem. We simulated 450 labelers, the number of labels workers labeled follow normal distribution with mean 20 and variance 10. We also generate 50 spammers who given wrong labels for objects with few labels on purpose to see the performance of our models. Finally, we get a dataset with 500 workers, 200 objects and about 10000 samples.

Table 2 presents the comparison results on the synthetic datasets. Overall, baseline methods are all better than MV. Figure 3 show the sample choosing process of SPGLAD-a and SPGLAD model. At the beginning of iterations, the number of samples chosen by SPGLAD is smaller than SPGLAD-a. Some samples which SPGLAD-a chose get low priori. After several iterations, SPGLAD chooses the same samples as SPGLAD-a and both of algorithms choose all samples at last.

Table 2. Error rate on the synthetic dataset

Method	Error rate
MV	0.276
D& S	0.264
3-Estimates	0.275
GLAD	0.258
SPGLAD-a	0.253
SPGLAD	**0.251**

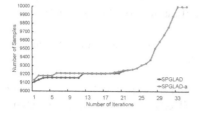

Fig. 3. Sample selection on synthetic dataset

Fig. 4. Error rate with different number of spammers

Table 3. Description of datasets

Dataset	Type	Workers	Objects	Samples
SRJ	3 choose 1	802	108	9352
Twitter-1k	2 choose 1	83	1000	5000
Sentiment	2 choose 1	143	500	10000
AdultContent	5 choose 1	825	11040	92721

We also compare GLAD, SPGLAD-a and SPGLAD by changing the number of spammers from 10 to 50. Figure 4 shows the error rate values of our models and GLAD model.

As we analyzed before, with the number of spammers grows, the difference between our models and the GLAD model becomes larger. Moreover, SPGLAD also behaves better than SPGLAD-a which proves the effectiveness of our prior distribution for w. Those differences prove that our model can learning datasets by choosing samples with easiness in a self-paced way.

5.3   Real-World Datasets

We further analyze our models on several real-world crowdsourcing datasets[3] including two-category and multi-categories. For multi-label models such as 3-

---

[3] Data are download from http://i.cs.hku.hk/~ydzheng2/crowd_survey/datasets.html.

Estimates and TruthFinder, we choose the label with highest probability as the category. Table 3 shows the description of each dataset.

For AdultContent dataset, we train our model with full dataset and use a subset with given ground truth to evaluate those models. This subset contains 333 objects with ground truth.

Table 4. Error rate on real-world datasets

Dataset	MV	D&S	3-Estimates	GLAD	SPGLAD-a	SPGLAD
SRJ	0.354	0.330	0.421	0.318	0.314	**0.312**
twitter-1k	0.324	**0.262**	0.377	0.282	0.274	0.274
Sentiment	0.060	0.082	0.092	0.056	0.047	**0.046**
AdultContent	0.205	0.219	0.208	0.197	0.188	**0.186**

The results are given in Table 4. SPGLAD get the best results in most datasets. For the Twitter-1k dataset, although our models perform worse than the D&S method, they still outperform GLAD. Due to Twitter-1k is pre-processed manually, there are few outliers in it. Since GLAD model does not get a high score, our model can not break through its upper bound. Table 4 also shows the comparison among GLAD, SPGLAD-a and SPGLAD. Our model behaves better than GLAD in all datasets. Particularly in AdultContent, our methods outperforms GLAD significantly.

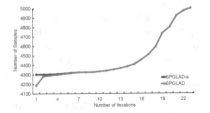

Fig. 5. Sample selection on Twitter-1k   **Fig. 6.** Sample selection on AdultContent

Figures 5 and 6 show the sample selection process in Twitter-1k and adult-Content datasets. For the Twitter-1k dataset, The sample selection process in SPGLAD behave similar to SPGLAD-a. However, the process behaves strikingly different in the AdultContent dataset. The reason is that there are many objects with few labels and workers given few labels in the AdultContent dataset. Thus, SPGLAD selects less samples than SPGLAD-a and increases slowly.

6 Conclusions

In this paper, we propose a self-paced GLAD model, which incorporates a self-paced learning process into traditional crowdsourcing quality control model. To avoid getting stuck on local optimum, the self-paced GLAD model defines the easiness of samples and optimize model with them. Moreover, we also provide priori which work as regularization to help model skip difficult samples at the beginning of iterations. Experiment results show SPGLAD model improves the performance compared with existing algorithms and the effectiveness of easiness w when choosing samples. It is easy to find models for rank or multi-label can also learning in a self-paced way. Combining our method with those algorithms is one promising direction for future research.

References

1. Bengio, Y., Louradour, J., Collobert, R., Weston, J.: Curriculum learning. In: Proceedings of the 26th Annual International Conference on Machine Learning, pp. 41–48. ACM (2009)
2. Dawid, A.P., Skene, A.M.: Maximum likelihood estimation of observer error-rates using the em algorithm. Appl. Stat. **28**, 20–28 (1979)
3. Fang, M., Yin, J., Tao, D.: Active learning for crowdsourcing using knowledge transfer. In: AAAI, pp. 1809–1815 (2014)
4. Galland, A., Abiteboul, S., Marian, A., Senellart, P.: Corroborating information from disagreeing views. In: Proceedings of the third ACM International Conference on Web Search and Data Mining, pp. 131–140. ACM (2010)
5. Karataev, E., Zadorozhny, V.: Adaptive social learning based on crowdsourcing. IEEE Trans. Learn. Technol. **10**(2), 128–139 (2016)
6. Kumar, M.P., Packer, B., Koller, D.: Self-paced learning for latent variable models. In: Advances in Neural Information Processing Systems, pp. 1189–1197 (2010)
7. Ma, F., Li, Y., Li, Q., Qiu, M., Gao, J., Zhi, S., Su, L., Zhao, B., Ji, H., Han, J.: Faitcrowd: fine grained truth discovery for crowdsourced data aggregation. In: Proceedings of the 21st ACM SIGKDD International Conference on Knowledge Discovery and Data Mining, pp. 745–754. ACM (2015)
8. Oyama, S., Baba, Y., Sakurai, Y., Kashima, H.: Accurate integration of crowdsourced labels using workers' self-reported confidence scores. In: Proceedings of the Twenty-Third International Joint Conference on Artificial Intelligence, pp. 2554–2560. AAAI Press (2013)
9. Venanzi, M., Guiver, J., Kazai, G., Kohli, P., Shokouhi, M.: Community-based bayesian aggregation models for crowdsourcing. In: the 23rd International Conference, pp. 155–164. ACM, New York (2014)
10. Welinder, P., Branson, S., Perona, P.: The multidimensional wisdom of crowds. In: Advances in Neural Information Processing Systems 23 (2010)
11. Whitehill, J., Wu, T.f., Bergsma, J., Movellan, J.R., Ruvolo, P.L.: Whose vote should count more: optimal integration of labels from labelers of unknown expertise. In: Advances in Neural Information Processing Systems, pp. 2035–2043 (2009)
12. Xu, C., Tao, D., Xu, C.: Multi-view self-paced learning for clustering. In: Proceedings of the 24th International Conference on Artificial Intelligence, pp. 3974–3980. AAAI Press (2015)

13. Yin, X., Han, J., Philip, S.Y.: Truth discovery with multiple conflicting information providers on the web. IEEE Trans. Knowl. Data Eng. **20**(6), 796–808 (2008)
14. Zhou, D., Liu, Q., Platt, J.C., Meek, C.: Aggregating ordinal labels from crowds by minimax conditional entropy. In: ICML, pp. 262–270 (2014)
15. Zhou, D., Basu, S., Mao, Y., Platt, J.C.: Learning from the wisdom of crowds by minimax entropy. In: Advances in Neural Information Processing Systems, pp. 2195–2203 (2012)

Author Index

Printed in the United States
By Bookmasters